TURN YOUR SUPERMARKET INTO A HEALTH FOOD STORE

THE BRAND NAME GUIDE TO SHOPPING FOR A BETTER DIET

LISA MESSINGER

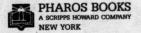

PHAROS BOOKS
A SCRIPPS HOWARD COMPANY
NEW YORK

Copyright © 1991 by Lisa Messinger.
All rights reserved. No part of this book may be reproduced in any form or by any means without written permission of the publishers.

First published in 1991.

Library of Congress Cataloging-in-Publication Data:
Messinger, Lisa, 1962–
    Turn your supermarket into a health food store : the brand name guide to shopping for a better diet / Lisa Messinger.
    p.   cm.
    Includes bibliographical references and index.
    ISBN 0-88687-620-6 : $6.95
    1. Marketing (Home economics)—United States. 2. Natural foods—United States.   3. Brand name products—United States.   I. Title.
TX356.M48   1991
641.3'1—dc20   91-15949   CIP

Printed in the United States of America

Interior design: Michael Mendelsohn of M 'N O
    Production Services, Inc.

Pharos Books
A Scripps Howard Company
200 Park Avenue
New York, N.Y. 10166

10   9   8   7   6   5   4   3   2   1

Pharos Books are available at special discounts on bulk purchases for sales promotions, premiums, fundraising or educational use. For details, contact the Special Sales Department, Pharos Books, 200 Park Avenue, New York, NY 10166

For Joel, a true and loving patron of my arts

CONTENTS

PART TWO
REPLACEMENT LISTINGS

CONTENTS..

ACKNOWLEDGMENTS

I would very much like to thank my editor, Shari Jee, who has been an inspiring and conscientious backer of and participant in this book. Thanks also to my agents Teresa Cavanaugh and Jean Naggar who were excited about and very interested in both me and this book. Gratitude to Rudy Shur for past and future publishing ventures, and for being a great friend. Thanks to the many supermarket chains who very graciously let me use their aisles for many hours as an essential "research library," as well as the *Antelope Valley Press*, a great base newspaper. Finally, thanks to my mother and father and supportive family members: Joel, Robert, Dalia, Regina, and Bea. And to a group of wonderful friends I grow prouder of each year: Doreen, Ilyce, Janine, Lisa, and Sandy.

PART ONE

HOW (AND WHY) TO TURN YOUR SUPERMARKET INTO A HEALTH FOOD STORE

1 : INTRODUCTION

J enny Silver, a bank manager, is strolling through her local supermarket. It takes her about an hour to shop for the week for herself and her urban-planner husband. As many of us do, she's throwing products that are "high fiber," "low cholesterol," and "all natural" into her shopping cart. She is tempted to buy the potato chips, but she and her husband are trying to eat better, so she regretfully passes them by.

Yet when Jenny writes her check for the cashier, she has lowered not only her bank balance but perhaps also her and her husband's good health, despite her good intentions.

That's because upon inspection Jenny's cart—filled with seemingly conscientious food choices—really proves to be filled with over a hundred different kinds of preservatives, chemicals, sugars, fats, and salts.

It is a common trap, but one that is surprisingly easy to avoid. Just by knowing how to make the most informed choices, Jenny could have quickly and easily been able to cut at least *90 percent* of those refined sugars, chemicals, additives, and preservatives, along with a hefty dose of fat and sodium, out of her diet without giving up one bit of taste.

She would not even have had to give up those potato chips—or lunch meat, hot dogs, even cakes or cookies.

That is where this book comes in. By using the principles outlined here and the extensive listings in Part Two (which give head-to-head comparisons of popular processed foods and their replacements), you can cut the possibly health-endangering ingredients in your pantry by a significant amount. And you can not only feel more full, be more energetic, and get all your nutrients; you can carve off unwanted pounds as well.

Of course, one way to make sure there are no additives in your food is to make everything yourself. But let's face it: Many of us are, like Jenny, too busy to make all our food fresh and from scratch. We rely more and more on packaged, often processed, convenience food. In 1990, a national food survey showed that convenience foods were the leader by far when it came to growth in product sales. What's interesting is that "guilt-free" foods and healthy snack foods followed closely behind. This just goes to show that most of us want it all—convenience and health benefits—when it comes to what we eat. We'll see how to read beyond health hype on food labels in Chapter 4.

As Jenny found, in trying to shop for health we may end up doing just the opposite. You may be a "Lean Cuisine Lady." Or you may believe Lynn Redgrave when she chomps on a Weight Watchers frozen pizza and chants "This is living!" You're eating processed convenience food, but you're keeping it light and calorie-conscious with dishes like these, right?

Unfortunately, we're being fooled. Did you know, for instance, that "no cholesterol" may mean that the product itself has no cholesterol but it may, in fact, be full of just the kind of oils that will cause your body to manufacture cholesterol? Did you know that an "all-natural" product can be filled with that natural cane product, refined sugar? Did you know that even if a product touts itself as "high-fiber," it may be chock-full of salt or sugar or preservatives or other things that cause laboratory rats to groan and won't bode well for you either? You may have chosen some of these foods because their manufacturers labeled them "light" or "healthy" but, even if some manufacturers don't, we should also be concerned about what goes into making them. We'll go over lots of the ingredients in "diet" foods that may surprise you in Chapter 3 when we look at the critical difference between most of those products and true health foods.

To start to become familiar with such manufacturer ploys, take a few minutes to go through your freezer, refrigerator, and pantry and read the fine print on the labels. Jot down all the chemicals, preservatives, sugars, fats, and other hard-to-pronounce ingredients listed in your foods. The sheer length of your list may be a great surprise.

Amazingly, in 1987, according to the Institute of Food Technologists, *7,855* new products that touted themselves as having some kind of beneficial nutritional modification showered the markets. These included 432 low- or reduced-calorie products, 159 that were labeled low in fat, 120 which were low in sugar, and 55 that bragged they were high in fiber. And this was before oat-bran mania had even entered the shopping picture!

With the advent of high-tech food technology, it is becoming a jungle out there in our supermarkets. In fact, of the 18,000 items in an average supermarket, *over 15,000* are processed.

Aside from the fresh meats, fruits, and vegetables in a market, just how are we supposed to find the well under 3,000 unprocessed—truly good for us—packaged products out of a sea of more than 18,000? And considering that there are over 3,000 food additives used in products, how can we find the select group of convenient, processed foods that contain no additives or preservatives?

As a 365-day-a-year active preventative/consumer/investigative health/nutrition columnist/reporter and food editor, I noticed that many packaged health foods were quietly moving into supermarkets from the strictly health food-store arena within the last few years. There are also a number of "normal" brand-name products that are truly healthful, additive-free foods, yet they're shelved right alongside their additive-packed competitors and, for the most part, don't even tout their benefits on their labels as much as the deceiving "health hype" products do. They're not technically "dietetic" foods, so they aren't stashed in their own special section of the supermarket.

In one major supermarket chain, a completely

healthy packaged pastry product is placed right next to the Pop Tarts. Completely whole-grain, high-fiber, unprocessed breads mingle with hard-to-tell-apart enriched, nutritionally bankrupt products. Nonfat, no-sugar, juice-sweetened yogurt is lost in a maze of sugar-, preservative-, fat-filled brands that are screaming to you from the shelf about how good they are for you. Interestingly, many supermarkets are not even promoting the fact that they may now be stocking foods once found only in health food stores. We'll take an in-depth look why in the next chapter.

It is now fairly easy to shop healthier, if only you knew these foods were out there and how to find them (and how to avoid health hype). The result of exhaustive research in supermarket chains nation-wide, this book offers a way to start putting healthier food on your table easily and immediately. Look up almost any of your favorite kind of processed or pack-aged food in the listings and you'll find a number of replacement foods that are just as fetchingly pack-aged, have no less taste, are not more expensive, and are truly good for you.

Do you feel like having ravioli or lasagna for din-ner? Look them up in the listing and you'll find them and comparable *health-promoting* replacements. Is it apple pie you're craving, or candy, cookies, chips, or pizza? Just look up any one of them and you'll find a natural, sugar-, caffeine-, additive-, preservative-free replacement. And if for some products there are no major brands available that totally fit that bill, we'll still let you know which one may be a much better replacement than the others.

Making just a few of the replacements listed can

make a significant difference; you can enjoy any foods without adding a drop of refined sugar or any artificial ingredient to your body. You can also cut down significantly on fat, especially saturated fat, and sodium. As a result, you'll actually feel better almost instantly, even drop some weight without trying, and make a difference in your long-term health.

We have been doing everything in our power to avoid cancer and heart disease. We are painfully aware of deadly statistics like the fact that 35 percent of all cancer deaths are attributed to poor dietary habits. The U.S. Department of Health and Human Services has noted that diet may play a role in 70 percent of all deaths.

Of the 3,000 additives used in our foods, some of them do not even have to be listed on food labels, so there is often no way for you to know when you or your family is ingesting them.

And you may not even be aware that pesky ailments like your headaches or lack of energy may be due to these ingredients. The replacements in this book show how you can rev up your body with "whole," unprocessed, delicious, convenient, high-energy fuel.

Obviously, we are going to keep purchasing convenient, packaged snacks and foods—they are the staple of many an individual's food life-style. According to *Snack Food Magazine*, in 1988 we spent about $25 billion just on snack foods. In 1986 our total snack dollars were divided this way: $7.4 billion on candy; $5.6 billion on cookies and crackers; $2.96 billion on potato chips; $1.46 billion on corn and tortilla chips; and $1.24 billion on packaged cakes and pies.

Turn Your Supermarket into a Health Food Store shows you how to point your food dollar in the direction of convenient, packaged foods that will actually improve your health, not rob you of it.

2 WHY YOUR SUPERMARKET MAY BE JUMPING ON THE HEALTH BANDWAGON WITHOUT TELLING YOU

A high-level executive with the Western division of a 527-store supermarket chain, who met his wife ten years ago when she was a checker and he was a clerk, wishes that his wife, now an accountant, would spend more time at the market where they met.

He's not sentimental or especially romantic, just practical.

"Cynthia runs out at least once a week to our local health food store," said Dave Hubbard,* an Albertsons markets executive, of his nutrition-concerned wife, who spends most of her leisure time working

---

* Name has been changed.

out at a nearby health club. "Even though she worked in our markets, she still goes out and pays about twice the price at a specialty health food store for the bulk of groceries for her and my daughter. She really doesn't know how much ours and other major supermarkets have changed. I tell her at this point she can get just about anything she buys at the health food store at the supermarket."

Cynthia isn't alone in not realizing the nutritional gold mine that awaits at her local supermarket. Since the trend of health foods moving into mainstream supermarkets is just beginning to explode, many consumers are not yet aware that there are now once-health food-store-only products available in virtually every aisle of their local supermarket. Since these products are often shelved right alongside others that *inaccurately* shout how nutritious they are, the truly healthful products may not be as easy to spot as you'd think. And, surprisingly—even though they could exploit them—many supermarket chains won't, don't, or simply can't make the consumer aware of a product's superior health qualities.

As recently as just a few years ago, almost all supermarkets relegated their meager supply of diet and health foods to a single aisle. That made the few products available easy enough for a shopper to find. But in most supermarket chains across the country "diet" foods are still residing in that same aisle while their upscale health food mates have moved on—in most cases leaving no forwarding address. Most markets now mainstream health or natural food products throughout their aisles. Because the number of health food products available has grown so dramatically, they outgrew their one aisle and now mingle with products throughout the supermarket.

That growth, of course, reflects consumer demand. But, unfortunately, even many of us demanding consumers are not necessarily able to tell at first glance the truly healthful food products from their "health hype" neighbors on the supermarket shelves.

But make no doubt about it, the products are moving in in full force. "Natural foods have reached the mass marketing stage, and soon supermarkets will be moving more volume than all the other natural foods businesses combined. In addition, some large food companies have jumped on the natural foods bandwagon and are now offering products without chemicals, preservatives, or additives. Nowadays, a consumer can find the same items in both a supermarket and a natural foods store," the editors of *The East West Journal* wrote in their *Shopper's Guide to Natural Foods*.

More and more healthier products are becoming available all over the country and to varied types of supermarket chains, but some top supermarket-chain executives need to catch up on the trend. "The Midwest is still a hard sell when it comes to health-type foods," one Western supermarket-chain manager commented. "They just don't seem to care as much there about those kinds of foods."

Rita Simmer—public communications manager for Super Valu, which owns eighty-three supermarkets including thirty-five Cub stores in Indiana, Illinois, Minnesota, and Wisconsin, among other states—couldn't disagree more.

"The central and Midwest parts of the country are

incredibly interested in these types of products," said Simmer, whose company is also a wholesaler to 2,800 supermarkets in thirty-three states. "The trend has grown even more in the last five to six years."

Supermarkets, with their aggressive advertising wars, are hardly bashful about tooting their own horns. If they are mainstreaming natural foods, why aren't they shouting down their aisles about it?

"Quite frankly, we did try to put 'headers' up on the aisles near the natural foods products that were once located in our diet aisle but now are integrated throughout the store," said Harland Polk, senior vice president of sales for the forty-nine-store Hughes market chain in Southern California. "But those headers just didn't work, mainly because of the physical makeup of the grocery aisle. We already had so many markers up for subgroups on each aisle that it was beginning to look like a telephone directory."

Those headers were not used, even though about four years ago (because, Polk said, "the category was simply exploding") Hughes mainstreamed health/natural food products throughout their stores and started purchasing them in larger and more varied quantities. There are very significant natural food presences on the chain's cereal, soup, salad dressing, candy, cookie, cracker—and many other—aisles.

There's another major reason aisle markers may not work for Hughes and other markets. It's true that natural foods have jumped to surrounding aisles from the "diet" shelf, but, now, more and more they are being joined by natural food versions of major, well-known brands. Even though the once-health food-store-only brands may be stocked together on a mainstream aisle, those natural *major* brands tend to be stocked right next to the original, not-so-natural, versions of their parent brands.

Ragú Homestyle spaghetti sauce, for example, which has no sugar or additives, is usually located alongside Ragú Old World Style 100% Natural and many other varieties of Ragú that contain sugar and corn syrup.

In addition, many huge food conglomerates are reacting to the explosion in natural foods sales by buying an existing health food company and expanding it.

Near East, a brand line based in Leominster, Mass., makes lots of hearty side-dish rice and other packaged products that fit the bill when it comes to making them natural/health foods. Although their package only identifies Near East and their Massachusetts plant, the company is now owned by Heinz, which is located in Pittsburgh. Hain Pure Food Company and the Hollywood brand, one of the biggest health food manufacturers in the country, was bought during the last decade by Pet Incorporated, the huge food conglomerate that also manufactures such products as Ac'cent flavor enhancer (MSG), and Sego diet drinks (which include many ingredients not found in health/natural foods products, although just because a huge food enterprise may now be the parent to a health food brand doesn't mean their quality is compromised). This can all add to the confusion, becoming one more vine added to the healthful versus unhealthful jungle our supermarkets have become.

A talk with Dan Thornton, brands marketing manager for San Francisco-based Tri Valley Growers, which is licensed by Nestlé to produce and distribute the Libby's canned fruit line, sheds more light on why even supermarket chains eager to stock natural products may have trouble making the presence of those products apparent to consumers.

Libby's has a number of products that contain no added sugar, preservatives, artificial flavors, or other such additives. The Libby's Lite brand of canned fruits, which are packed in fruit-juice concentrates rather than sugar or syrup, stands out over many other canned-fruit "lite" brands. Or does it?

Thornton says that the main competitor for Libby's Lite in supermarket canned-fruit aisles across the nation is Del Monte Lite. This seems logical. However, Del Monte Lite canned fruits contain sugar, although they simply say "in extra light syrup" on their labels. The peach versions of these two lites do have the same calories per serving: fifty. Ironically, Del Monte also has *another* canned-fruit line called Fruit Naturals that, because it is packed in juice and has no sugar, is much closer to the Libby's Lite line—but with a mere *ten* more calories per serving! Many people, though, might consider it more important to avoid refined sugar than those ten extra calories. This is one of many cases where *lite* on one product can mean something quite different on another product.

Maybe your supermarket still has that specially marked "diet" aisle. Many do.

"When we mainstreamed the natural foods products, we kept the rest of the diet food together where it had always been. We think most of the customers shopping in the diet section are there because of a particular medical need," said Polk of Hughes markets.

Do you have a particular medical need? Or are you simply trying to eat in an overall healthful way that helps you avoid developing that medical need in the first place? The fact that these "diet" aisles are now mainly for specially prescribed eating plans is becoming an important trend to note all over the country. If you're still shopping in that one "diet" aisle, thinking that it is your supermarket's prime spot for healthful fare—which many consumers do—you may be severely limiting your options when it comes to buying the healthiest food available in your supermarket.

What you may be getting is a "no-sodium" product that is, indeed, missing the sodium but loaded with artificial colors or flavors or sugar. Or you may get a "no sugar" product that's full of salt. Natural foods are healthful across the board. Special "diet" foods (look at some of those sugar-free hard candies in your supermarket's "diet" aisle and what it takes to make them) may just limit one ingredient while throwing caution to the wind when it comes to what else is in the product. Look closely, for instance, at many of the high-protein weight-loss drinks and drink mixes available on most supermarket "diet" aisles and you are likely to spot a laundry list of multisyllable synthetic ingredients that might even make a laboratory rat look for the nearest exit.

Kroger markets, the Cincinnati-based company that includes such other market chains as Dillon and King Supers, is the second-largest supermarket chain in the country. The Kroger stores alone number over 1,200 and virtually blanket the country in eighteen states between Texas and Virginia.

In many of the Kroger stores, shoppers will see the same type of diet aisle that Hughes sports in California, according to Dianne Vesio in Kroger's corporate affairs department. However, Kroger for the most part has also mainstreamed the health/natural food products that once shared the diet aisle. Kroger, like many chains, gives individual stores or regions much autonomy, so you might shop in one Kroger and find health/natural products in a special gourmet section and in another Kroger find the same kinds of product in a special health food section, and in yet another Kroger find no such special sections but see the health/natural products throughout the store.

Many supermarket chains are also displaying lots of small "health-related" notes in each aisle. Beware! Just like a suiter trying to win your affections by only showing you his best side, these shelf markers—a new and growing trend—may be so bent on wooing you that they become deceptive without even trying.

For example:

- At Hughes (similar to many other Southern California markets) you'll see Nutritags, which point out foods that fit FDA guidelines.
- Safeway, the nation's third largest supermarket chain, with about 1,100 stores up and down the West Coast and in Alaska, Hawaii, and Canada, has mainstreamed most once-health food-shelf-only products throughout their stores, according to public affairs chief Brian Dow-

ling. They also have shelf tags throughout the store reflecting their praised Nutrition Awareness Program.

- Byerly's, an upscale Minnesota supermarket chain, has had tags pointing out low-sodium and low-calorie foods for years.

These tags—nutritional love notes from your supermarket to you—are popping up all over the country. They are your supermarket's way of letting you know they are aware of the phenomenal health revolution being waged by consumers. However, the problem is that generally the tags only concentrate on one aspect of the product. One tag will say a product is low-fat. But what else is in it? How much salt is in it? Is it all artificial or does it actually have some natural ingredients? I've seen low-fat supermarket shelf tags in front of jams and flavored gelatins. True, these and many other foods are low-fat. But many of those jams have sugar and additives. The "lite" versions have artificial sweeteners and other fillers. Unfortunately, so far, there have been no tags in supermarkets that take into account the *entire product*.

Polk of Hughes and Dowling of Safeway, like many other supermarket executives, point out that they're trying to help consumers with programs such as these "nutritional" shelf tags, but, they say, ultimately it is the manufacturer's responsibility to keep us informed about health benefits.

Unfortunately, because many manufacturers make inflated or incomplete claims, that ultimately means the responsibility falls to us.

3 | THE CRITICAL DIFFERENCE BETWEEN "DIET" FOOD AND YOUR NEW HEALTHY ALTERNATIVES

"**U**nfortunately, some of my friends who really care about their health and are trying to shop healthfully—like most people—see *lite* or *low-calorie* or *low-fat* on a product and they're virtually blinded by the word," said Helene Peltz, comptroller of twenty-six Key Food stores that comprise the largest group of independently owned supermarkets in the New York metropolitan area. "They grab the product and run with it and think it's some kind of health and nutrition panacea. Fortunately, because of my work for a group of supermarkets, I've learned some of the tricks of the trade and know that's just not the case. Believe me, with what I've learned, I read *the ingredients.* I know those other words on the label are no indication of a health panacea."

Whether it's people like Peltz's well-off, well-educated friends or many of the consumers in the Key Food stores she works for (a number of which are located in economically depressed areas of the city, but still report growing sales of "lite" and "reduced-calorie" products) there seems to be almost universal acceptance of these popular foods.

Many of us who are concerned with weight control have opened our arms wide to this ever-increasing array of "calorie-reduced" products. Unfortunately, however, for our overall health as well as our actual diet success, we often did not look behind the claims on the fronts of these packages. "Low calorie," "Dietetic," "Under 300 calories." This is what we read and what we understandably bought.

And bought we have. In 1990, the Calorie Control Council (CCC), an international association of manufacturers of low-calorie and diet foods and beverages, found that two out of every three American adult men and women consume light products. And, CCC found, we consume these products, on average, four times per week.

However, as Peltz and those who have been opting for "natural" foods over "diet" foods are all too aware, many such light products are filled with sugars, additives, preservatives, chemicals, and artificial ingredients. Do the majority of consumers realize this and simply put up with it in order to eat a food that is low in calories or fat or sodium? That, unfortunately, is not the case. The CCC survey found that nine out of ten light-product consumers say the main reason they eat light foods is "to stay in better overall health." Weight loss was much lower down on their list of reasons. In fact, a 1989 CCC survey of more than ninety million consumers of low-calorie foods found that fewer than half were actually dieting.

Of course, packaged convenience foods are here to stay. We're too busy not to use them. However, you can easily and quickly avoid the chemicals, preservatives, and artificial ingredients in these "diet" products that may be playing havoc with your weight, your mood, and your health.

But should we really be concerned about these popular foods? What's the problem?

Well, out of 202 brands of low-calorie beverages and foods, for example, 84 percent were shown to have as their ingredients additives of concern to all people, according to extensive studies reported by Nicholas Freydberg and Willis Gortner, former director of the Human Nutrition Research Division of the USDA. Ninety-one percent of 100 regular frozen dinners, pizza, and pot pies proved to have additives of concern.

It's clear why we try to shop for foods that we feel are more healthful, whether we're on target or not. After all, study after study has shown that what we eat affects our health. Cancer. Heart disease. As much as we aerobicize, jog, or bicycle, these are the things we are staring in the face down the line if we don't get a grip on what we eat.

Shouldn't we trust food manufacturers or the government—the Food and Drug Administration (FDA), which oversees what additives are used in foods—about the foods, whether light or regular, that we buy in our supermarkets? To a certain extent, of course we should be confident. However, there are some key points to be aware of which form the basis of why more and more people choose to avoid foods prepared with additives and preservatives.

Additives in foods are usually used in such small amounts that perhaps you think you really don't eat much of them. However, Michael Jacobson, executive director of the Center for Science in the Public Interest, cites studies showing that the average American consumes about five pounds of additives a year. When you think about the small amount of additives used in most foods, you can see just how many additives you would have to be eating—and how often—to add up to five pounds. When you include sugar (which is the food-processing industry's most used additive and an abundant ingredient in many "diet" foods), that number jumps to 135 pounds per year.

The FDA declares some additives Generally Recognized as Safe (GRAS). Other additives they declare GRAS but note that further study is needed. Ruth Winter's *A Consumer's Dictionary of Food Additives* lists many additives as "GRAS status continues while tests are being completed and evaluated."

Does it make you secure to know that the government actually *never* feels confident enough about any additive to give it a fully clean bill of health? Information from the Food Safety and Inspection Service (FSIS) of the United States Department of Agriculture (USDA) shows that "Additives are never given permanent approval. FDA and FSIS continually review the safety of approved additives to determine if approvals should be modified or withdrawn."

Of course, you don't receive information that an additive is generally recognized as safe but still judged to need further testing when you see such an additive listed on a product label. Why fill yourself and your family with additives when many still need more testing and it is fairly easy to avoid them? And, most important, why consume additives that today may be declared GRAS but that in two or ten or twenty or more years are thrown off the GRAS list and out of the food supply because their true status as a carcinogen finally becomes known? You may end up with twenty years of the additive under your belt, in your bloodstream, or clogged in an artery before its true dangers are discovered or acknowledged by the FDA.

And this has happened. Cyclamate, a widely used sugar substitute through 1970, was shown to possibly cause bladder cancer and was eventually banned from products. But, as Jacobson reported, even fifteen years later the company that sold cyclamate was still asking the FDA to allow its use.

Xylitol, another sugar substitute that was touted as a great way to avoid tooth decay, was used in Care-Free gum, LifeSavers, and other products in the 1970s. It was approved for use by the FDA in 1963 but studies later found that it seemed to promote bladder tumors in laboratory animals. American companies stopped using xylitol. According to the Center for Science in the Public Interest, an FDA official said that "it had to be conceded that xylitol appeared to induce tumors in a dose-related manner in both rats and mice." However, although the FDA proposed banning xylitol, it never completed the action. Some candies imported from Finland (where the additive originated) are available in U.S. markets and still contain the additive.

Among many others, there's also a very recent example of an additive we've been ingesting for decades that the FDA just recently banned. In January 1990 the FDA announced the delisting of FD&C Red Lake No. 3 (an artificial coloring) in foods, drugs, or cosmetics.

Studies showed that high dosages of FD&C No. 3 have triggered thyroid changes that could cause cancer. "FD&C Red No. 3 is a proven carcinogen. The FDA has taken twenty-nine years to make a final decision," reported attorney William Schultz of Public Citizen (an organization founded by Ralph Nader) to the media when the ban was imposed.

And yet, while some uses of an additive like FD&C Red No. 3 may be banned, we still may be ingesting the questionable additive while final steps are taken by the FDA.

"The recent ban involves only the provisional approval of the food color in lake [powdered] form and does not yet disapprove 'permanently' listed uses of the food dye form in ingested drugs and foods (e.g., maraschino cherries). However, the lengthy legal process to delist all applications will be initiated by FDA," *Food Processing: The Magazine of the Food Industry* recently advised its readers.

It's not as if there are no natural alternatives to additives like Red Dye No. 3—or virtually any other chemically derived additive. Japanese researchers, for example, recently introduced in the United States a coloring derived from red cabbage. Since it is made from natural vegetable juice, it doesn't even need FDA approval. It is already being used in salad dressing, juice, and hard candy. It also may soon be used in tomato and barbecue sauces, pudding, and yogurt. Food-trend magazines are predicting the red cabbage extract will be a major food ingredient in the next decade.

Besides eating maraschino cherries, gelatin, dyed pistachio nuts (all of which also contain Red Dye No. 3) or other foods that may contain additives the FDA is trying to get rid of, many experts point out that there may be serious implications to ingesting the rainbow of additives and preservatives available that the FDA has not even considered.

Although the FDA may look into the effect a single additive has on a test animal, many of us (especially when we eat "diet" or "lite" foods) consume many different additives every day, many within a given meal. How do these additives act together? This is a scary scenario that, as we munch away on thousands of additives a year, no one has yet fully studied. And because of the sheer number of additives and possible combinations, adequate studies might not even be possible.

Dr. Arnold Fox, a well-known Beverly Hills cardiologist and former professor of medicine at the University of California at Irvine, articulated this widely held concern in *Immune for Life*, a book he wrote with his son Barry: "We don't know what happens when the chemicals get together inside your body. Chemical A in your ice cream may be relatively harmless by itself. So might Chemical B in your fast food french fries. But what happens when the two chemicals meet in your bloodstream or liver? Do they ignore each other? Do they combine? Does A convert B into a more dangerous form?"

This kind of combined exposure to chemicals also recently made news when an environmental group, U.S. Public Interest Research Group, questioned Environmental Protection Agency (EPA) standards.

A report from the group stated that the government should halt all use of cancer-causing chemicals in food since there is no way of knowing how many different substances a person consumes. The accumulated exposure has not been studied. A few years ago, the agency said, EPA published a list of cancer-causing substances in foods, but this made no note of how the different substances might work together in our bodies.

And what about additives that the government knows the effect of upon our bodies, but because the public is so addicted to them—the way people are with cigarettes—would probably never consider cutting from the food supply? These additives don't carry warnings about their true nature on product labels. How much do you know, for instance, about caffeine?

Many of us—especially dieters—consume lots of caffeine in coffee, tea, and diet sodas. No diet label would say "Caffeine is not just hazardous to the health of your pancreas, it is classified medically as a poison." That came from a treatise on caffeine, *Nutritional Self-Defense*, by medical researcher Frances Sheridan Goulart. Her report goes on to say

"[Caffeine] is a nitrogenous organic compound of the alkaloid family whose chemical name is trimethyl-xanthine. Morphine and strychnine belong to the same family." It has been shown that animals that have had large injections of caffeine will be dead within minutes. Caffeine injected into human muscles can cause paralysis.

In addition to a "poison" like caffeine, what is actually in some of these "lite" or "diet" products? It is easy to get caught up in just seeing the seductive words on the front of a package rather than studying the terribly small print stashed on the side or the back.

On the front of the label of Mrs. Butterworth's Lite, for example, we are told that it is a reduced-calorie syrup with no artificial sweeteners, and that two tablespoons contain 60 calories instead of the 110 of regular syrup.

So what are the ingredients used to make this product instead of regular syrup, which just comes from a tree? Sugar syrup, water, corn syrup, natural and artificial flavors, cellulose and xanthan and algi-nate gums, salt, caramel color, butter (butterfat removed), sorbic acid (preservative), sodium citrate, sodium acid pyrophosphate, sodium benzoate (preservative), and fumic acid.

Besides the preservatives and artificial ingredients in this product, remember that, in addition to "salt," anytime you see an ingredient preceded by the word *sodium*, you are ingesting more sodium. In Mrs. Butterworth's Lite, therefore, you are getting four separate doses of sodium.

Many of us rely for lunch or dinner on low-calorie

frozen entrées—to the tune of $460 million in 1989. Yet besides calories, there are other considerations when it comes to these products. What about sodium? Some are loaded with it. And what about fat? It's fat that counts when we are trying to lose weight. A national food technologist's study showed that low-calorie frozen entrées differed in fat content by as much as 250 percent! And this wasn't obvious, either. A turkey and fish entrée were significantly higher in fat, for example, than a beef product. And what about what is used to make these meals?

For health, and especially when we're dieting, it's important to know the difference between saturated and other types of fat. All fats have both saturated and unsaturated (fatty acids) fat. Animal products are the main sources of saturated fats. Saturated fats are much more likely than other fats—poly- or monoun-saturated fats—to cause your body to manufacture cholesterol, which can lead to heart disease.

Why not try this: The next time you see a Weight Watchers Deluxe Combination Pizza, count the number of ingredients on the back of the label.

Of the *60 ingredients* in this product, there are listings like mononitrate, b-cysteine, low-moisture part-skim mozzarella cheese substitute (which includes a number of ingredients of its own, none of which is cheese), sodium aluminum, trisodium phosphate, artificial color, artificial flavor, zinc oxide, and cyanocabalamin.

Chemists and scientists are concocting "foods" like this for you to eat, surely a trend that will grow in the future, They create "foods" that appeal to the taste buds—but logic would deny that they could be significant providers of nutrition when they are chock-full of these additives.

Of course, these products go through testing in order to be approved by the FDA. NutraSweet, for example, went through more than a hundred tests over eight years before it was approved. Many health groups still question the safety of chemically, scientifically derived products like NutraSweet. And, of course, since something like NutraSweet was only introduced into the marketplace in 1981, there is no way to know its possible long-term effects. The FDA seconds that opinion, since, as noted earlier, it will never grant permanent approval to any additive but rather keeps the door open for further testing.

But although many of the additives in "lite" or "diet" foods are not permanently approved or may be GRAS with a disclaimer that further testing is still needed, they can quickly infiltrate the food supply. For example, even though NutraSweet (which was originally discovered accidentally by a pharmaceutical company developing an ulcer drug) has only been in the marketplace for a relatively short while, it is already in over 150 products worldwide. It is the world's number-one-selling sugar substitute and enjoys annual sales of over $800 million. Scientists are feverishly working to get NutraSweet into every possible product, and the company's chairman says, eventually to replace sugar completely.

Commercials for NutraSweet tell us that it is made up of amino acids—components of protein—just like a banana or other natural food. But when was the last time you saw a banana being painstakingly put together in a lab by chemists in white coats and long robot computer-automated arms? That's what the inside of the NutraSweet labs look like. Aspartame, called NutraSweet under patent arrangement in this country, is a methyl ester of the peptides phenylalanine and aspartic acid and therefore is metabolized as a protein. Very little resemblance to a banana or any other natural food!

Another new addition to the "lite" foods market is "fake fats" as well as the products they are beginning to spawn. Simplesse fat substitute is made by the makers of NutraSweet. It is an ingredient in Simple Pleasures Frozen Dairy Desserts, and the company recently announced it will be making it available to other manufacturers—much as it did with NutraSweet—for use in their products.

There are many other fat substitutes under development or review. For example:

- DDM (dialkyl dihexadecylmalonate), under development by Frito-Lay, is a synthetic fat and may be appropriate for fried foods and snacks.
- EPG (esterified propoxylated glycerol), being developed by ARCO Chemical Company, is noncaloric and can substitute for fat or oil.
- Modified Protein Texturizers, Kraft's addition to the fake-fat market, is similar to Simplesse, as its process begins with proteins that have been changed in physical form.
- Olestra is a calorie-free fat substitute being developed by Procter and Gamble; the FDA is reviewing it.

- TATCA (trialkoxytricarballylate), CPC International's entry into the fat-substitute race, has no calories and is an oil-like compound.

Soon we may be able to eat completely synthetic "lite" foods for every meal. However, some prominent health organizations are warning against that. The Mayo Clinic recently made an appeal in its *Nutrition Letter*:

> This is an era of high-tech food, but that doesn't mean you should eat indiscriminately and rely on artificial processing to keep you healthy. A proper diet involves more than leaving "bad things" out. It means taking "good things" in.
> The proliferation of substitutes may soon mean you can eat a completely synthetic meal, from appetizer to dessert. Yet the long-range health effects of these products are unknown. Questions also remain about how artificial foods mix with medications and other substances in the body.

However, some large food manufacturers would argue that additives and preservatives are necessary and must be in products to prevent spoilage or make them creamier or easier to pour. Some foods may require these ingredients, but, precisely because of public concern and awareness, enough major manufacturers have begun joining the small ones who have always been natural to prove that, in most cases, it simply cannot be argued to be a necessity.

Would you, for instance, have to think twice about buying Orville Redenbacher's Gourmet Natural Flavor Microwave Popping Corn or Newman's Own All Natural Flavor Microwave Popping Corn? Almost all the other brands of microwave popcorn available—including Pop Secret, Planters Premium Select, and Jolly Time—have added "to protect flavor" questionable preservatives like BHA, BHT, and TBHQ (a particularly troublesome ingredient that contains petroleum-derived butane and took much pushing by manufacturers before FDA approval. As little as a five-gram ingestion has caused death; one gram resulted in collapse, nausea, vomiting, delirium, and a sense of suffocation). The Redenbacher and Newman's Own brands do not have these preservatives. Are you going to be any less happy with those brands? Will the flavor be noticeably different? Most consumers who buy those products wouldn't think so.

Unfortunately, you, like much of the population, may have grown so used to the additives, chemicals, and preservatives in "lite" and "diet" products—as well as the rest of the food supply—that you may not realize just what toll they are taking on your whole system.

You may have become tolerant to drugs like caffeine and all of these other substances, but once you start replacing even just a few foods, you will probably notice an immediate and marked difference in how you feel on a day-to-day basis. You'll sleep better. You'll have more energy. You will simply feel better physically. And you'll never have to go near a so-called diet food again.

4 | HOW TO READ BEYOND HEALTH HYPE

I n a hurry to finish shopping and get home to her two children, Mary Joseph grabbed a large can of Hawaiian Punch from the supermarket shelf. She was glad to notice the red banner on the product that read "7 natural fruit juices. Full day's supply of vitamin C." As she dropped the can into her cart, she also noticed that it stated it had no caffeine and was very low in sodium.

Not until she had poured her children some of the Hawaiian Punch did she look more closely at the label and notice what was actually in the product. The first three ingredients (meaning they were used in higher concentrations than the fruit juice ingredients that followed) were water, corn syrup, and sugar. Since the product had touted its "7 *natural* fruit juices," Mary was also especially surprised to see among the fine print such ingredients as dextrin, a flavor carrier that is used in, among other things, matches, fireworks, and industrial dyes; artificial color; artificial flavor; and ethyl maltol, a synthetic flavor enhancer produced from the hydrocarbon contained in alcohol.

Bob Gerard stopped off at his local supermarket at the end of his daily jog. He thought he'd grab a quick drink. His pick was Kern's Strawberry Banana Nectar. Like Mary Joseph, Bob was in a rush, but he noticed a few things on the label. First of all, there was the photo of the luscious-looking fruits on the front of the can. He also noticed that the label prominently stated that the nectar had "no artificial flavors or preservatives added." Bob didn't even feel he really needed to examine the Kern's label because he had always considered the product—as many consumers did—a health food brand. He was more sure of that when he read on the label that "Kern's fruit nectars are made from the whole fruit—not just juice—so every delicious sip is filled with genuine fruit goodness."

Bob didn't realize until he was outside the store and enjoying that first delicious sip how true that statement was; Kern's nectars are, in fact, "not just juice." Bob read the fine print and saw that the two main ingredients of the beverage were water and high-fructose corn syrup. Another surprise guest on the list was artificial color.

Bob and Mary are just two of the millions of consumers who say they are beginning to feel they should have a library card issued by their local supermarket. Because food manufacturers are aware of our growing interest in health, there are more and more statements being made on food labels, and so more and more to read on every label of every product we buy.

Until 1987, when the Reagan administration discontinued an eighty-one-year-old ban on such claims, only special diet products were allowed to make nutritional claims.

Without the ban, however, food manufacturers began playing dirty with our tremendous interest in health. Virtually every product in the supermarket—from soup to nuts, cakes to frozen casseroles—has filled every available inch of space on its label with some sort of nutritional claim.

Some shoppers have become cynics. "There are no totally healthful foods available in major supermarkets," I overheard a disgusted woman mumble as she checked out with a full cart. That's simply not true. Even with a sea of manufacturers screaming nutritional contradictions at you, there are some extremely simple tenets you can follow that will immediately cut through the hoopla and hype and bring you to the nutritional heart of the matter.

If you realize that some of even the most logical-sounding claims may not be true, you're already ahead of the game.

But maybe you're *not* a cynic when it comes to deciphering food labels. Maybe you think that it couldn't be simpler to tell which products are full of hot air (as well as lots of additives) even though they boldly proclaim nutritional superiority on their label. My many days of research in supermarkets, however (as well as interviews with quite a few health-concerned shoppers), made it clear to me that there are many products doing such a good job of hyping themselves as healthful that they would keep even the most nutritionally savvy on their toes.

KNOW WHAT TERMS REALLY MEAN
....

Therefore, before we look at some of the simple steps you can take to quickly find products that are refined sugar-, caffeine-, preservative-, additive-, and chemical-free, let's wade through some common nutrition information minefields found on many product labels.

First, however, you should know that not all products are required to carry nutrition information on their labels. Some manufacturers do so voluntarily, but they are not required to do so unless they make a nutritional claim or the product has been enriched (the process of replacing nutrients lost during processing) or fortified (adding nutrients not present in the natural state of the food). Currently, only about 55 percent of packaged products carry nutritional listings. This will be changing in the future due to new labeling laws, which we will discuss in a moment.

However, even when they do give nutritional information, beware. The same word may have different meanings on different labels.

- Light ("lite") foods are near the top of all new product introductions. But *light* can mean a variety of things. It can mean that a product is lower in calories than its original version. It can also simply mean that it is lighter in taste, texture, color, fat, cholesterol, or sodium. Suggested new labeling procedures may eventually result in a standard definition for terms like *lite*, but most nutrition experts agree that it will be years before any such changes are fully in effect. That's virtually millions of bites you and your family will take while labeling information is still sketchy.

- "No-salt" or "salt-free." A product labeled *no-salt* may have other sources of sodium. The American Dietetic Association warns that there are over seventy different sodium compounds used in food processing, and whether a product says "no salt" or not, if those compounds are present, sodium will still be added to your diet. This is why, as we'll stress later, it is so important to look at the *nutrition per serving* listings on a food label. The sodium milligrams listed there will tell the true story.

Incidentally, although here we mention the American Dietetic Association, and elsewhere we give a nod to the California Dietetic Association, basic nutritional guidelines are an area where, fortunately, almost all major organizations agree. From the offices of the Surgeon General to the dietary guidelines of the USDA to the materials distributed by the American Diabetes Association, the American Heart Association, and the American Cancer Society, there is widespread agreement: eat a variety of *fresh* foods. Cut down on fat. Increase fruit and vegetable consumption (for cancer prevention). Use dairy products to increase calcium intake. Use sugar and alcohol moderately. What you'll notice missing in the literature from any of the organizations, however, is encouragement about eating any additive or preservative.

Nutritionists recommend a limit of 3,000 milligrams of sodium per day. To put this into perspective, we must first be aware that just one teaspoon of salt has 2,300 milligrams. But since most of us never sit down to read our morning paper and to enjoy a teaspoonful of salt, what does this mean in terms of the foods we actually eat? Well, if your lunch included two slices of Eckrich salami, you'd be ingesting 1,200 milligrams of sodium. If dinner included a serving of Campbell's Home Cookin' Country Vegetable Soup, that would add another 1,070 milligrams. The Weight Watchers Lasagna entrée you might have with your soup would represent another 990 milligrams to your sodium count. At a total of 3,260 milligrams of sodium, that puts you over the recommended level after eating only three foods!

Look for any ingredient with the word *sodium* in it to clue you to the fact that the food is probably high in sodium. Even though these may be there as preservatives or additives rather than flavor enhancers, they still add sodium to your diet. The salami, for instance, besides salt, lists sodium nitrite. The soup sports salt and monosodium glutamate.

Other sodium label terms, besides *no-salt* or *salt-free* on a label do carry particular meaning. *Sodium-free* means that the product has less than 5 milligrams of sodium in a serving.

Low-sodium has 140 milligrams of sodium or less

in a serving. *Very low-sodium* has 35 milligrams of sodium or less in a serving. *Reduced-sodium* means that the usual level of sodium in a product has been reduced by at least 75 percent.

- "No refined sugar." The product may have no refined sugar, but may boast other processed sugars like high-fructose corn syrup. Also, although products list their ingredients by descending order according to weight, this system can also be misleading when it comes to sugar, sodium, or other ingredients of interest to the health-conscious. A manufacturer may list one ingredient as sugar, another as high-fructose corn syrup, and a third as brown sugar or molasses. Therefore they are distributed throughout the ingredient list, but if all sugars were listed together (as the Center for Science in the Public Interest has suggested), sugar would then be listed first as the product's primary ingredient.
- "High fiber." There is not yet any standard definition of this term. As syndicated nutrition writer Lorna Sass has noted, "Your definition of high (fiber) may be someone else's definition of low." Nutritionists recommend 20 to 25 grams of fiber per day. Foods considered good sources of fiber usually contain three or more grams of dietary fiber per serving. Many products claim they are good sources of fiber even though there is barely any bran or fiber in a serving. The FDA just recently sent letters to six more companies warning them to re-

move what they called just such "unsubstantiated claims."

- "Low cholesterol" and "low fat." These terms can be very misleading since there are no standard definitions. *Low fat* is only defined in the dairy aisle, where it means that milk with less than 2 percent fat is considered low-fat.

We've seen a lot of complex mathematical ways to determine how much of a percentage of fat a food contains. One quicker way to calculate this is to think that for every hundred calories of a product you eat, ideally, look on the label and, there should be no more than three grams of fat. Therefore, if a label reads that a serving of food has 200 calories, there should be no more than six grams of fat listed for that serving.

Nutritionists want you to have no more than 30 percent of your daily calories from fat. As for cholesterol, the American Heart Association and other health organizations suggest no more than 300 milligrams per day.

However, knowing how much fat or cholesterol (found only in products of animal and not plant origin) experts want us to eat may not help when we come across the sea of hype on many products. "Ingredient claims can be more confusing than helpful. Perhaps the best example is the plethora of products marked 'cholesterol-free,' " noted Jean Mayer, president of Tufts University, and Jeanne Goldberg in their syndicated nutrition column. "But are you better off buying a food labeled this way? Not necessarily. The catch is that the product beside it on the shelf that lacks a cholesterol-free tag ... also may contain no cholesterol."

Then, there are also manufacturers promoting cholesterol-free versions of foods (say, mayonnaises) that barely had any cholesterol to begin with. Although they have introduced low-cholesterol versions, for example, Kraft and Hellmann's mayonnaises in their regular versions only contain 5 milligrams of cholesterol. Other products, like peanut butters, also shout on their packages that they are cholesterol-free when they never even had any cholesterol in the first place.

When it comes to fat claims on products, consumers can also be easily duped. Many products are now claiming things like "85 percent fat-free" or "95 percent fat-free." That sounds pretty good, doesn't it? Well, many people don't realize that these descriptions refer to the weight of a fat in a food, not fat calories. The potentially misleading fact is that fat—although high in calories—actually weighs very little.

"Fat labeling is the most confusing," American Dietetic Association president Nancy Wellman has said, "especially when terms such as '95 percent fat-free' or '85 percent lean' are used." Wellman points out that a turkey frank labeled "80 percent fat free" actually has 72 percent of its calories from fat.

- Ingredients. Many manufacturers throw in little apologies or explanations along with their ingredient lists. After a particularly chemical-sounding ingredient, for example, a manufacturer might add in parentheses "to preserve freshness."

Or they will take great pains to explain their culinary (although artificial) choices to you. Perhaps they'll slip in after artificial/chemical ingredients the words "promotes tartness" or "assures creaminess." But there are plenty of versions of these products that are just as tart or creamy that don't rely on such artificial, chemically based tactics. This is just one more way many manufacturers are trying to cloud the nutritional issues and manipulate us as we scan their labels.

Take note, though, that sometimes ingredients that sound a little "fishy" may actually be acceptable. The difference between the terms "natural" and "natural flavorings" highlights this.

Although the word "natural" when used on food labels is in that murky, controversial area that can mean a number of things, when the term "natural flavorings" is used, there is a standard Food and Drug Administration (FDA) regulation that must be followed.

The FDA's Federal Code of Regulations Section 101.22 declares that "natural flavoring" may be applied to "the essential oil, oleoresin (a naturally occurring mixture of an oil and resin, as the exudate from pine trees), essence or extractive, protein hydrolysate, distillate or any product of roasting, heating or enzymolysis which contains the flavoring constituents derived from a spice, fruit or fruit juice, vegetable or vegetable juice, edible yeast, herb, bark, root, leaf or similar plant material, meat, seafood, poultry, eggs, dairy products or fermentation products thereof whose significant function in food is flavoring rather than nutritional."

Therefore, if you are sensitive to dairy products, you might want to keep in mind that a product including natural flavorings may include dairy product derivatives. Some monosodium glutamate (MSG) experts also point out that protein hydrolysate (or hydrolyzed vegetable protein, as it is also called) may contain up to 20 percent MSG. Those who feel they are sensitive to MSG should be aware that some natural flavorings may contain small amounts of it.

WON'T NEW LABEL GUIDELINES HELP CLEAR THE CONFUSION?

···

After all of this talk about how confused many current labels can make us, won't the new FDA guidelines we've been hearing about come to the rescue and make sense of everything?

The guidelines, which are in the long process of being implemented, are, of course, a major step. No sweeping food label changes have been made since 1973, when vitamin and mineral content on labels was the main issue. In November 1990, President Bush signed the Nutrition Labeling Act of 1990 into law. The law is a directive to the FDA and under it, eventually almost all food and beverages will be required to have nutritional labeling (rather than the current 55 percent).

The new labels will add information about fats and saturated fats, cholesterol, and dietary fiber. However, because many manufacturers are already keenly aware of our interest in health, these issues have already been covered voluntarily on many labels. There may eventually be standards for health claims like "light" or "natural," as there are already for "low-sodium" and "calorie-reduced."

A number of people cheer the new changes, but some nutrition experts say that the changes may add too many components and just add to the confusion.

James Tillotson, a Tufts University professor and director of that school's Food Policy Institute, has said he even thinks there's a danger in telling consumers too much on a label. Tillotson, who amid the 1990 debate about new labeling held a symposium on the subject, has said he thinks that a label should announce calories, carbohydrates, protein, saturated and unsaturated fat, and percentage of calories from fat.

"Other than that," he told the Chicago *Tribune*, "I'm not sure it doesn't become an academic exercise."

Bearing out Tillotson's prediction that confusion may be the result of new labeling guidelines are the first products to hit the markets boasting that they are following new FDA-proposed guidelines.

These products follow the proposed listing of Daily Reference Values. These let consumers know, for example, how one of the product's 13 grams of fat per half pizza serving stack up to the 75 grams of fat the FDA says is suitable for a healthy diet. It does the same for saturated fat. This assumes consumers will be keeping track daily of exactly how many grams of nutrients they are eating. There are also the same type of listings for cholesterol, carbohydrates, fiber, and sodium. Where is protein? Why wouldn't we be counting protein in a scenario like this? Also, although we're to assume it wouldn't be healthful to go over the amount of fat for a healthful diet, what about the 25 grams of fiber listed? Will consumers start making that their cut-off point, too, even though fiber is generally considered a good substance that it would be better to *increase* in the diet than to decrease?

Interestingly, the new DRVs are based, across the board, on eating a diet of 2,350 calories! How many women attempting to watch or maintain their weight are eating 2,350 calories? Many people watching their weight try to consume only 1,000 or 1,200 calories per day. How can advice based on this one high-caloric assumption be of help to individuals with varying needs?

The American Dietetic Association has questioned this caloric issue. In commenting about the National Academy of Sciences' tables of recommended energy intake of 2,350 calories daily, Christine Lewis, section chief of the FDA's Division of Nutrition, told the ADA, "That's more than the 1,800 to 2,100 calories some groups have traditionally used as a reference intake, so some people think it's on the high side." And, again, for dieters (many of whom are *more* interested than anyone else in nutrition labels in the first place), the new labeling (if based on a diet of 2,350 calories) may become useless.

The problem, of course, is that none of the new legislation deals with *what is actually in the foods we eat*. Many studies have shown that most consumers only look at a food label for about ten seconds before buying a product. (That's why manufacturers make claims so large and colorful—hoping you won't get to the tiny print regarding ingredients and nutrients and such.) With all the old and new information to appear on labels, there is still absolutely no guarantee that consumers will spend their ten seconds or so reading ingredients.

And, you'll note, this act is labeled a nutrition law. Most additives (excluding refined sugar, which provides lots of calories) add absolutely no nutritive value to foods. They are not increasing the calories (although many increase sodium levels), or the grams of protein, carbohydrates, or fat. They are foreign substances and, in many cases, of questionable safety.

And in any event it will still be quite a few years before all the new labeling regulations—whether they actually prove useful or not—see fruition in our supermarket aisles.

And there is already a whole new wave of health hype beginning based on the new labels!

Totino's, for example, a frozen pizza made by Pillsbury, recently sent press kits to daily newspaper food editors boasting of being the first product to use FDA-proposed nutrition labeling information. There was a lot said about how Totino's now has leaner meat and how they're following the new guidelines.

There is even a Totino's booklet called "Healthful Hints!" available from the Pillsbury Consumer Center. But there was still no clear word sent with this information on exactly what is in the product. However, anyone who looks at their label in the supermarket knows that, leaner meat or not, there's still a laundry list of ingredients in Totino's, including artificial color and other additives. Since Totino's (which uses the new confusing DRVs we've been discussing) is an indication of how new guidelines may be presented on labels to the public, it seems we may be in for more—rather than less—confusion.

WHEN IT COMES TO LABELS, YOU CAN LOSE THE CONFUSION AND GAIN KNOWLEDGE

Although we all know how confusing current product labels can be—and we've seen that the new labels may not do much to clear up that confusion—the real key to cutting through all of this hype and hoopla is simpler than almost anyone could imagine. The real key is to trick the labels, rather than letting them trick you: Don't read them.

Don't read labels? Well, for the most part. Ignore all claims, which vary widely from product to product, and read only two parts of the label that appear on virtually every product: the *ingredient listing* and the *nutritional information per serving*. This information will be on both current and new nutrition labels. Some current labels already do, and all of the new ones will list fiber and cholesterol.

Instead of looking at those "cholesterol-free" or other colorful banners (not to mention contests, giveaways, and so on), on the front, take just ten seconds or so to flip it around and read the fine print first. Believe it or not, this will give you all the information most informed shoppers need to drastically reduce their intake of enriched products, refined sugar, additives, chemicals, and preservatives.

This may seem obvious and logical, but I am constantly surprised that most people giving mainstream "nutritional" advice never suggest it.

For example, in the beginning of 1990, a major publisher announced with much fanfare a first-of-its-kind book, compiled by a respected registered dietitian. It promised "nutritional information" for all "lite" and other modified foods on the market. Lots of products are listed, broken down in every imaginable way, but—to many a reader's surprise—not an ingredient anywhere.

Similarly, as a food editor of a daily newspaper, I just recently was sent a "pitch" and samples for a column from a major syndicate. The column, also by a dietitian, was promised to be *the* place for readers to look to find all pertinent information regarding food labels. The author even compared and rated products head-to-head. Again, however, ingredient listings were not a part of her nutritional criteria.

ONCE YOU READ BEYOND THE HEALTH HYPE, WHAT KINDS OF THINGS ARE YOU LOOKING FOR?

People who have shopped for years in special health food stores can attest to how wonderful (and often trim) a natural food diet can almost immediately make you feel. The basis of what they've been doing can easily be emulated by you in your own supermarket.

For all the benefits, applying the tenets of a simplified program of natural foods shopping is very easy. If you adhere to some of the following steps, you'll be well on your way to getting expensive health food-store results at a supermarket price.

Today's shoppers are busy. We don't have time to study product labels for hours on end. This system is a speed-reading method of healthful shopping. The method is based much more on what you are trying to avoid than on what you are necessarily looking for.

First, flip a product around and skip all the hype and focus immediately on the list of ingredients.

Quickly scan the ingredient list. If you see enriched or fortified products, consider moving on. This only means the product is not generally whole-grain; part of it has been removed, which is why it has had to be enriched. Everyone from C. Everett

Koop, the former Surgeon General, with his landmark suggestions on nutrition, to every corner nutritionist seems to agree that whole grains—which include all fibrous parts—are much better for you than anything enriched.

If you spot sugar, artificial sweeteners, corn syrup, or high-fructose corn syrup as ingredients, consider moving on. Look for products that are fruit juice-sweetened. Honey and fructose (natural fruit sugar) are acceptable choices since they are in their natural, more nutrient-dense state and are unrefined. Rice syrup is also a natural sweetener.

Some manufacturers will try to tell you that all sugars (refined fructose, honey, and the like) are alike. All sugars are basically digested alike (although sugar from fruit and honey are digested a bit more slowly)—quickly, which is why they translate to quick energy. However, much of the similarity ends there.

We already know about the dangers of artificial sweeteners. Products containing saccharine already bear warnings that the sweetener may have caused cancer in laboratory animals. We talked about the artificial way NutraSweet is made and some of its possible health concerns in Chapter 3.

But what about refined sugar? Lots of manufacturers put large lettering on their packages claiming "all natural." A close look at the ingredients, however, shows that some of those products are mainly sugar. The chemical formula for sugar is $C_{12}H_{22}O_{11}$. Multiple chemical processing of the sugar cane or beet (those are the natural substances the manufacturers are referring to) produces sugar. That process, however, also removes all fiber and protein, both of which made up 90 percent of the original sugar plant. This is truly what is meant by "empty calories" (there are 2,500 calories in a pound of sugar). And yet refined sugar is by far the top additive in packaged foods today, with the average person consuming 130 pounds of it a year.

What's the difference between sugar and honey? William Dufty explains the facts well in his best-seller *Sugar Blues,* which was hailed by both consumers and medical experts:

> Pure is a favorite adjective of the sugar pushers because it means one thing to the chemists and another thing to the ordinary mortals. When honey is labeled pure, this means that it is in its natural state (stolen directly from the bees who made it), no adulteration with sucrose to stretch it and no harmful chemical residues which men have sprayed on the flowers. It does not mean the honey is free from (beneficial) minerals like iodine, iron, calcium, phosphorus, or multiple vitamins. So effective is the purification process which sugar cane and beets undergo in the refineries, that sugar ends up as chemically pure as the morphine and heroin a chemist has on his laboratory shelves. What nutritional virtue this abstract chemical purity represents, the sugar pushers never tell us.

As you speed-read through product ingredient lists, you'll probably also notice a lot of listings for high-fructose corn syrup (not to be thought of as the same thing as fructose, which is unadulterated fruit sugar). Again, we recommend that when you see this ingredient—if your goal is a health food diet—you consider moving on to another product.

High-fructose corn syrup is used as a cheap substitute for refined sugar. Almost all soft drinks and many other packaged food products use it. According to the Mayo Clinic's report on high-fructose corn syrup in its *Nutrition Letter*, the additive gained wide acceptance when sugar prices rose between 1974 and 1980. High-fructose corn syrup now makes up half of all sugar consumption, according to Mayo.

High-fructose corn syrup contains fructose, while regular corn syrup, also used as a sweetener, does not. High-fructose corn syrup is made from corn by food companies that chemically change glucose in cornstarch to fructose. Quite a difference from a product that is sweetened by, say, 100 percent grape juice!

Once you know what you are looking for when it comes to sweeteners, the rest of the speed-reading natural food shopping course involves spotting any artificial, chemical, or preservative ingredient on the list. We've already seen what a tenuous existence many of these additives lead—being declared safe by the FDA only to have that approval withdrawn later. Or how there have never been any tests on how all of the three thousand food additives we eat—even if they're determined safe by themselves—interact when they meet other chemically derived additives in our bodies.

Within product ingredient lists, artificial color and flavor are listed as such. Often, a manufacturer will insert "preservative" following such an ingredient. Other additives usually stand out like a sore thumb, since they are usually listed among real foods but don't sound like they are real foods. For example, it's easy to see the standouts in ingredient listings reading: "wheat, corn, TBHQ" or "wheat, corn, myristaldehyde." If you see artificial ingredients, chemicals, or preservatives listed, move on to other products. If you want to avoid caffeine, you'll see that right away in the ingredient list, too, and you can also move on. And, of course, you can use the listings in the back of this book.

Just by looking at ingredient listings, you'll find lots of products that are whole/natural foods. You may also find lots of foods that are good replacements because even though they may have sugar or some other additive, they are not filled with artificial ingredients or preservatives like other foods in their category. Once you find them, you can then check their other attributes by employing step two of our speed health shopping tips: Look at the nutrition per serving on the label. Quickly scan calorie, fat, and sodium totals. Eliminate any product that seems very high (based on the levels we went over earlier) in any category.

As simple as this elimination process sounds, if you follow it, you'll have an excellent chance of cutting about 90 percent of the refined sugar, chemicals, preservatives, and caffeine out of your and your family's diet. It's a short course to making an immediate marked improvement.

5 HOW TURNING YOUR SUPERMARKET INTO A HEALTH FOOD STORE CAN HELP YOU LOSE WEIGHT

S arah Mason says she finds it hard to understand why she doesn't seem to be losing much weight on her diet or why she often gets headaches, or feels depressed or tired.

Although she can't give an exact number, this thirty-four-year-old executive secretary is sure she has been on at least a hundred weight-loss plans over the last fifteen years.

Surprisingly, Sarah's 101st diet, as well as many of ours, may not be working precisely because we are eating processed, packaged, artificial "diet" products. New information reveals that sweeteners—artificial or low-calorie or not—may make us crave even more sweets. And the chemicals and preservatives and sodium we get along with our "diet" foods may, in fact, be in large part responsible for our headaches or draggy feelings while dieting.

Sheila Winters, like Sarah, is also a veteran dieter. However, she has managed to step off the diet roller coaster. One day recently Sheila could not believe her eyes. When she looked down at her bathroom scale, she weighed fifteen pounds less than she had just six weeks earlier.

Unlike Sarah, this time Sheila had not gone on any calorie-restricted diet. She had not stopped eating most of her favorite foods.

Jason Winters, Sheila's husband, didn't go on a diet either. Yet, he's dropped a size in clothing and ten pounds he wasn't even trying to lose.

Although the Winters didn't go on a diet, restrict the amount of food that they ate, or stop eating their favorite dishes, they had, in fact, done something. They had inadvertently turned their supermarket into a health food store.

Sheila had finally decided to throw in the towel and give up on diets. After much reading and study on health, her resolution was to simply try to eat more healthfully. She decided to cut most refined sugar, most enriched products, artificial ingredients, chemicals, and preservatives from her diet. Weary of feeling tired and hungry much of the time, Sheila thought her new eating habits might make her feel better—but she didn't realize she would see such a quick and significant weight drop.

Sheila and Jason (who had joined his wife in the quest for a healthier diet) are just two of a growing number of people who attest to the magic of a natural food eating plan. The "magic" is that the partakers often feel they are not eating less food and not giving up their favorite foods, but, still—whether they've unsuccessfully tried other diets or not—the pounds just seem to roll away. Sarah, unfortunately, is still a part of an even larger group: those who eat packaged "diet" foods and constantly bob up and down as yo-yo dieters.

Before we look into just why natural food eating habits can have such a positive effect on weight loss, it's perhaps just as important to briefly study why some of the "weight loss" choices we may be making now may be providing little result.

When Sheila, for example, decided to cut refined sugar from her diet, she didn't think she was eating much of it in the first place. After all, she had been peppering her menus with "diet" foods for years, and tried to stay away from "sweets."

Like many of us, however, Sheila didn't realize just how many foods are "sweets" to one degree or another and may be helping us add unwanted pounds. Many people, in fact, are eating their weight in sugar every year. As we reported earlier, the Mayo Clinic reports that consumption of sugar per person in the United States is 130 pounds.

That number must reflect all the people who feast on ice cream and candy and cake, many people would say. However, according to the Center for Science in the Public Interest, sugar is the leading food additive *across the board* in all processed, packaged products, far outdistancing any of the other three thousand additives used.

When frequent dieters like Sheila, for example,

pop a Lean Cuisine frozen lasagna into their oven, most are probably not even considering the fact that sugars would be a player in a food used for weight control. But in addition to many other ingredients, sugar makes an appearance three separate times in this entrée: In addition to being added to the overall product, sugar is an ingredient in the "mushroom base" and is also added to the product in the form of sugar-cane syrup.

And as much as these products tout themselves, there has never been any conclusive proof that calorie-reduced products are actually helpful when it comes to losing weight. According to a 1989 report by the Institute of Food Technologists' Expert Panel on Food Safety and Nutrition, "Low calorie foods, ingredients and analogs cannot offer quick fixes or serve as magic bullets to weight loss or control." It went on to say "that so far there is no evidence that the proliferation of these foods has had any effect on how fat Americans are." In fact, although 80 million Americans—about one in three—say they follow weight-control diets, obesity is still rapidly increasing rather than going down.

And as far as artificial sweeteners go, the data on weight changes in 78,694 women who were involved in a twenty-year study (between 1968 and 1988) on mortality with the American Cancer Society actually showed that women who used artificial sweeteners were more likely to *gain* weight than those who did not.

Lots of weight-concerned consumers drink a number of cans of diet soda every day. Many think the soda will depress their appetite or fill them up when they might have eaten a high-calorie food. In addition to the fact that many of these beverages contain additives, acids, and caffeine, there have also been studies which have shown they may even encourage weight gain.

Scientists at the University of Pennsylvania-based Monell Chemical Senses Center, the world's leading independent research institute that studies taste, during the last five years, noted some interesting findings when it came to diet soda. The studies indicated that drinking diet soda could make imbibers hungrier. The results showed that the hunger was a fairly short-term effect after drinking the soda. But when people are downing three or four or more servings of diet soda a day, a burst of hunger after each could certainly add up to lots of snack breaks.

Another new addition to the "diet"-food market are "fake fats" and the products they are beginning to spawn. Simplesse fat substitute, made by the makers of NutraSweet, is an ingredient in Simple Pleasures Frozen Dairy Desserts. Dreyer's American Dream frozen dairy dessert is 99 percent fat-free. Kraft has introduced a similar line from its Knudsen division. Sara Lee and Hostess have also used technology recently to bring virtually fat-free versions of their products to supermarkets.

However, the California Dietetic Association put out an alert after Simplesse was approved. They were hoping to warn eager dieters:

> [Simplesse] is not the miracle ingredient one might imagine where calories are concerned. Dieters should beware: the caloric savings are not as substantial as weight watchers may first be

led to believe. A four-ounce serving of an ice cream-like product made with the fat substitute contains 120 calories. Regular ice cream is about 150 calories per serving.

According to the Mayo Clinic, when dieters eat noncaloric food they simply do not lose weight. Research subjects always made up the deficit caused by those foods by eating even larger amounts of something else.

The Mayo Clinic *Nutrition Letter* also warned readers about fat substitutes: "We think it's too early to count on worry-free foods. In fact, the whole subject of food substitutes needs more study."

The first step to making the transition to a natural food diet for weight loss is not to believe that you must be perfect. If you want to try to cut out refined sugar and all preservatives, chemicals, additives, and enriched foods from your diet, that is noble, and you will undoubtedly reap rewards.

However, one of the benefits of eating natural foods for weight loss is that even if you just start substituting them for the occasional meal, snack, or dessert, you will also notice results. Your biggest surprise might come from, say, only cutting refined sugar from your diet. Since we eat so much sugar without realizing it, if you consciously avoid products that list refined sugars, you'll probably drop weight without even counting calories.

Stephen Blauer, former director of the Hippocrates Health Institute in Boston, author of *The Juicing Book* and co-author of *The Macrobiotic Way,* has often seen the results a natural food diet can quickly deliver. Blauer, who deals quite a bit with macrobiotic (grain-based) eating plans, said that he has told people the difference between a regular processed food diet and a natural food one is often a right-off-the-bat weight loss of about fifteen pounds.

"But won't I be eating more calories if I give up my low-calorie packaged food for all-natural, non-calorie-reduced, supermarket products?" is the question many people ask.

The truth is that you will probably eat less because natural foods tend to fill us up faster and leave a longer feeling of fullness.

Lots of studies have shown this, but a 1988 one from Yale University provides a graphic example of how the most natural, least-refined foods are the best choices when it comes to weight loss.

The researchers had twenty-four women and men between ages twenty-two and fifty drink lemonade sweetened with either fructose (natural fruit sugar) or refined sugar. About thirty minutes later the subjects were offered a buffet lunch. Those who had drunk the fructose beverage consumed an average of 30 percent fewer calories and chose less fatty foods than the other test participants. The drink that included refined sugar stimulated the subjects' appetites. The researchers reported that they were unsure of the precise reason fructose curbs the appetite, but that it might be related to the fact that it is metabolized more slowly than other sugars.

Another reason you feel more full when eating natural foods is because you are no longer eating a lot of fillers or additives. You are, say, eating more whole grains within a product (this adds the bulk of fiber, which nutritionists recommend for successful weight-loss diets), which can give you more sustained energy over a longer period. And if you're not eating sugar or caffeine, you won't experience any of those sugar or caffeine "rushes" followed by "crashes" so often experienced by frequent dieters.

Your body will also be running on higher-quality fuel. Therefore you will probably not want to "fuel up" as much as you used to.

Dr. Harvey Ross, a Los Angeles nutritionist and psychiatrist who has written and co-authored a number of popular books such as *Fighting Depression* and *The Mood Control Diet*, recommends natural, whole-food diets for weight loss to hundreds of clients.

"When you eat natural foods," he said, "you may feel better or lose weight because instead of having to deal with all kinds of additives, your body is just being filled with quality ingredients, nutrients, all of which are used productively by your system. Nutrients fill your body's needs, and, therefore, your body sends you less, if any, signals in the form of cravings."

Once your system is cleared of products (some of them drugs, poisons, and stimulants) that manipulate how you feel—like sugar, artificial sweeteners, and caffeine—you probably will no longer have cravings for unhealthful or "junk" foods that cause you to gain weight. Your body will start to ask you mainly for natural food.

Of course, not all "natural" foods are low-calorie, low-fat, and low-sodium (however, many more of them are than additive-filled packaged foods are).

The trick is, by looking at the ingredient listings and the nutrition per serving on the labels, to find some of the many that are.

There are lots of foods in your supermarket that promote health *and* weight loss. That's the point. We shouldn't be eating one set of foods to lose weight and another to promote health. There are lots of products that do both. Find them in Part Two of this book and in your neighborhood supermarket, and there's a good chance you'll find yourself as trim—and healthy—as you'd like to be.

PART TWO

REPLACEMENT LISTINGS

6 ALL YOUR FAVORITE PACKAGED, PROCESSED SUPERMARKET FOODS AND WHAT TO EAT INSTEAD

W elcome to a world of select products available in supermarkets that contain no refined sugar, no preservatives, no artificial ingredients, chemicals, caffeine, or other additives. Most of the replacement products listed also are not enriched, and rely instead on whole grains. There are also lots of products listed that may contain sugar or an additive or two, but are not chock-full of the artificial ingredients and preservatives that might make up most of the other foods in their categories.

Welcome also to a world of great tastes. Like a cookbook author who tests her recipes, I have tasted many of the products listed. And, indeed, I regularly fill my shopping cart with them. One guideline for these products was that they were to taste as good as any additive-filled version of the same food. In fact, because of their usually superior ingredients, most taste much, much better than products with lots of additives.

Take a quick look at how painless and tasty replacement shopping can be:

- Would your family notice if you brought home Ragú 100% Natural Pizza Sauce rather than Ragú Pizza Quick Sauce, or Mott's Natural Apple Sauce instead of Original Tree Top Apple Sauce? Probably not, since the sets of products taste virtually identical, but you will have eliminated the added sugar.

- Would your husband bat an eye if he found Kellogg's Nutri-Grain Wheat flakes in your pantry instead of Wheaties? Most people probably wouldn't mind, especially if they knew it meant adding whole grain and at the same time eliminating refined sugar, corn syrup, calcium carbonate, calcium chloride, trisodium phosphate, and BHT from their cereal bowls.

- Would your tortilla chip taste any different if it were dipped in La Victoria Salsa Picante Sauce rather than Pace Picante Salsa Sauce? The only difference is that with Pace it was bathing in a sauce that contained no traces of the modified food starch, sugar, and the preservative benzoate of soda in La Victoria.

You'll find products in the listings grouped by category, much as you would in your supermarket. There are head-to-head comparisons between additive-containing products and those that are better choices. You'll see ingredients listed for the two comparison products, as well as nutrition per serving and other brand-name products that should also be replaced or that may be suitable as healthful replacements.

Products—whether those suggested for replacement or the replacements themselves—that are particularly high in sodium or fat are marked with an asterisk. Guidelines of the American Dietetic Association, which considers over 400 milligrams a high sodium count for a food serving when people are trying to eat healthfully, were used.

When available, nutrition per serving listings were taken directly from a product's label or, when not listed, obtained directly from the manufacturer. A listing of the country's most popular national brands, in some cases, was also consulted.

You'll find no favoritism in the listings. A company may find itself listed in one category as an additive offender and in another category praised for one of its other products. In some categories, it's as easy to improve your diet as picking another of the same company's brands.

Although virtually all of the products profiled are national, there are a few points you might want to keep in mind. For example, we listed some breads in order to show comparisons of what to look for. However, with a little speed health-label reading, most of you will find local companies that supply your supermarkets; that will add variety to our healthful bread listings. The same may be the case with dairy products. Some will be national, others delivered by local dairies.

Most of these brands (whether offenders or replacements) are those you've often spent your food dollar on: Hunt's, Ragú, Kellogg's, Campbell's, Libby's. However, one of the theories behind this book is that brands from companies once only available in health food stores are now quickly and quietly moving into mainstream supermarkets. Because of the sea of health hype out there, they may be getting lost in a crowd of imposters. To keep you informed about these and other exceptional health brands from smaller companies that may soon become major health players, we've put a "be on the lookout for" tag beside them in the listings. These tags will note exceptional health products that are just beginning to make their presence known in supermarkets nationwide.

Some of these once-health food-store-only brands you've probably heard of. As we mentioned in Chapter 2, Hain products and its Hollywood brand have recently been bought by the giant food conglomerate Pet in St. Louis. They are two of the biggest health food brands sold in supermarkets throughout the country.

There's a good chance you are also familiar with Irwindale, California-based Health Valley, Inc., the country's largest health food company, which makes over two hundred products. Although Health Valley has been in business for more than twenty years, the real explosion in mainstream supermarket sales only occurred three or four years ago when, according to Harry Urist, one of the company's directors, the national oat-bran craze hit. Urist said it was then that supermarkets started really increasing Health Valley orders, orders that have just kept growing.

In addition to health giants like Health Valley and Hain, lots of small, independent companies are adding exceptionally healthful products to supermarkets all over the country every week. You may not have heard of them yet. But their products can help anyone trying to follow a health food diet in a supermarket world.

Just Delicious Gourmet Foods, which recently introduced a line of natural/healthful soup mixes to supermarkets nationally, is a case in point. They are a small company and offer such innovative no-sugar, no-additive soup mixes as Spicy Chicken Vegetable, Champagne Bean, Black Bean Chili, Gourmet Minestrone, and Champagne Red Lentil.

However, according to Dan Smith, the company's vice president, it is tough to stand out in a sea of imposters who say they are doing just what you have always done. At one point, for example, Campbell's was sent a cease-and-desist letter by the FDA because the label implied that some of its soups (many of which contain monosodium glutamate, sugar, and other additives) were good sources of calcium. Actually, it was the milk that was added to the soups that provided the calcium.

"We don't want to be stocked in a special health food section," Just Delicious' Smith said. "We try to get in the mainstream right next to all the other soups. But it's difficult. Many supermarket chains charge companies large amounts of money for shelf placement. We've even won awards with our packaging, but everyone else is claiming on their label to be healthful, when our products really are."

Some of the following listings—those that bear our BE ON THE LOOKOUT FOR tags—will introduce you to new guys (like Just Delicious) on the supermarket aisle block. But mainly the listings will provide you important information about healthful products from your all-time favorite major companies.

Get familiar with these replacement brands and you'll be on your way to achieving health food-store quality while shopping in your local supermarket.

CONDIMENTS
(Salad dressing; dips; mayonnaise; ketchup; mustard; pickles; barbecue sauce; salsa; sweeteners)

SALAD DRESSING: VINAIGRETTE/ITALIAN

PRODUCT: Wish-Bone Lite Classic Dijon Vinaigrette

> INGREDIENTS: Water, vinegar, soybean oil, Dijon mustard, lemon juice, sugar, salt, dehydrated onion, spices, dehydrated garlic, natural flavors, dehydrated red bell pepper, potassium sorbate, calcium disodium EDTA, xanthan gum, artificial flavor, annatto.

> NUTRITION PER SERVING: ½ fluid ounce (1 tbsp.) serving; 30 calories; 0 g protein; 1 g carbohydrate; 3 g fat; 180 mg sodium.

PRODUCTS TO REPLACE: Most major brands, including: Hidden Valley Ranch Italian; Hidden Valley Ranch Take Heart Italian; Kraft Free Italian Nonfat; Kraft House Italian; Kraft Zesty Italian; Newman's Own Reduced-Calorie Light Italian; Seven Seas Viva Italian; Weight Watchers Italian-style.

REPLACEMENT: Newman's Own Olive Oil and Vinegar Dressing

INGREDIENTS: Olive oil, soybean oil, red wine vinegar, lemon juice, spices, salt, fresh onion and fresh garlic.

NUTRITION PER SERVING: 1 tbsp. serving; 80 calories; less than 1 g protein; less than 1 g carbohydrate; 9 g fat; 80 mg sodium.

OTHER REPLACEMENTS: Hain Naturals Creamy Italian; Hollywood Classic Creamy Italian; Marie's Italian (refrigerated) Dressing.

BE ON THE LOOKOUT FOR: Cardini's dressings; Mrs. Kinney's Italian Dressing.

SALAD DRESSING: CREAMY DRESSINGS

PRODUCT: Wish-Bone Ranch Dressing

INGREDIENTS: Partially hydrogenated soybean oil, water, vinegar, maltodextrin, salt, sugar, dehydrated egg yolk, xanthan gum, polysorbate 60, dehydrated buttermilk, onion, monosodium glutamate, dehydrated garlic, lactic acid, potassium sorbate, sodium benzoate, calcium disodium EDTA, natural and artificial flavors, dehydrated spices, disodium guanylate, disodium inosinate.

NUTRITION PER SERVING: 1 tbsp. serving; 80 calories; 0 g protein; 1 g carbohydrate; 8 g fat; 160 mg sodium.

PRODUCTS TO REPLACE: Most major brands, including: Hidden Valley Ranch Take Heart Ranch; Kraft Free French Catalina; Kraft Free Ranch; Kraft Rancher's Choice Ranch Reduced-Calorie; Kraft Thousand Island; Richard Simmons' Salad Spray Roma Cheese; Seven Seas Viva Ranch Light; Wish-Bone Chunky Blue Cheese; Wish-Bone French; Wish-Bone Russian.

REPLACEMENT: Hain Naturals Old Fashioned Buttermilk

INGREDIENTS: Soy oil, water, grain vinegar, sour cream solids, eggs, cultured buttermilk solids, honey, salt, soy sauce (water, wheat, soybeans, salt), spices, vegetable gum, lemon juice concentrate, onion powder, garlic powder, natural flavorings.

NUTRITION PER SERVING: 1 tbsp. serving; 70 calories; 0 g protein; 0 g carbohydrate; 7 g fat; 100 mg sodium.

OTHER REPLACEMENTS: Hain Naturals Thousand Island; Marie's Blue Cheese (refrigerated) Dressing.

DIPS

PRODUCT: Frito-Lay's Jalapeño Cheese Dip

INGREDIENTS: Water, cheddar cheese (milk, cheese culture, salt, enzymes, calcium chloride), vegetable oil (contains one or more of the following: partially hydrogenated soybean oil or partially hydrogenated cottonseed oil), modified food starch, buttermilk, jalapeño peppers, tomatoes, cornstarch, disodium phosphate, natural cheese flavor, yeast, salt, spices, onion, monosodium glutamate, acetic acid, sodium citrate, artificial color, mono- and diglycerides, garlic, sodium benzoate, citric acid, calcium chloride.

NUTRITION PER SERVING: 1 ounce serving; 45 calories; 1 g protein; 3 g carbohydrate; 3 g fat; 310 mg sodium.

PRODUCTS TO REPLACE: Most major brands, including: Frito-Lay's Bean; Frito-Lay's French Onion.

REPLACEMENT: Padrinos Bean and Salsa Dip

INGREDIENTS: Pinto beans, water, tomato paste, fresh onions, fructose, salt, fresh jalapeños, onion powder, peppers, garlic, spices.

NUTRITION PER SERVING: 1 ounce serving; 30 calories; 2 g protein; 5 g carbohydrates; less than one g fat; 160 mg sodium.

OTHER REPLACEMENTS: Amigos Bean; Eagle Mild Bean; Hain Mexican; Hain Onion; Hain Onion Bean; Hain Taco.

BE ON THE LOOKOUT FOR: Nasoya Vegi-Dip Creamy Dill; Nasoya Vegi-Dip French Onion.

MAYONNAISE

PRODUCT: Kraft Real Mayonnaise

INGREDIENTS: Soybean oil, eggs, vinegar, water, egg yolks, salt, sugar, lemon juice concentrate, paprika, dried garlic, dried onion, calcium disodium EDTA, natural flavor.

NUTRITION PER SERVING: 1 tbsp. serving; 100 calories; 0 g protein; 0 g carbohydrate; 12 g fat; 70 mg sodium.

PRODUCTS TO REPLACE: Most major brands, including: Best Foods Light; Best Foods Real Mayonnaise; Hellmann's Real Mayonnaise; Kraft Light; Light n' Lively Reduced-calorie Mayonnaise; Miracle Whip Cholesterol Free; Miracle Whip Light; Miracle Whip; Weight Watchers Reduced-Calorie Mayonnaise.

REPLACEMENT: Hain Safflower Mayonnaise

INGREDIENTS: Safflower oil, water, whole eggs, honey, grain vinegar, spice, salt, egg yolks, lemon juice concentrate, extractives of paprika.

NUTRITION PER SERVING: 1 tbsp. serving; 110 calories; 0 g protein; 0 g carbohydrates; 12 g fat; 70 mg sodium.

OTHER REPLACEMENTS: Blue Plate Mayonnaise (has sugar, but no artificial ingredients or preservatives); Hollywood Natural Safflower Mayonnaise.

KETCHUP

Most ketchups are fairly good health bets since they don't have artificial ingredients or preservatives. The one additive most do have is corn syrup. The examples here give you a choice for a replacement that uses honey rather than corn syrup.

PRODUCT: Heinz Tomato Ketchup

INGREDIENTS: Tomato paste, tomatoes, distilled vinegar, corn syrup, salt, onion powder, spice, natural flavoring.

NUTRITION PER SERVING: 1 tbsp. serving; 18 calories; less than 1 g protein; 4 g carbohydrate; 1 g fat; 180 mg sodium.

PRODUCTS TO REPLACE: Most major brands, including: Heinz Low Sodium Lite; Hunt's; Del Monte: Springfield.

REPLACEMENT: Hain Naturals Catsup

INGREDIENTS: Tomato paste, water, honey, grain vinegar, onion powder, garlic powder.

NUTRITION PER SERVING: 1 tbsp. serving; 16 calories; 0 g protein; 4 g carbohydrate; 0 g fat; 15 mg sodium.

BE ON THE LOOKOUT FOR: Westbrae Natural Fruit-Sweetened Catsup.

MUSTARD

We skip a listing for mustard because all major brands are good health bets. Mustard, which is usually made from vinegar, water, mustard seed, salt, and spices, is a health food that's always been in your supermarket. It's a good condiment to choose over sugary products (like ketchup) when possible.

PICKLES

Most major brands of pickles have a preservative. If you'd like to avoid the sugar also present in many brands, go with our replacement below or most most major dill pickle brands.

PRODUCT: Heinz Sweet Cucumber Slices

INGREDIENTS: Cucumbers, distilled vinegar, high fructose corn syrup, salt, dehydrated onions, spices, calcium chloride, natural flavoring, FD&C yellow No. 5, polysorbate 80.

NUTRITION PER SERVING: 1 ounce serving; 25 calories; 0 g protein; 6 g carbohydrate; 0 g fat; 169 mg. sodium.

PRODUCTS TO REPLACE: Most major gherkin and sweet cucumber slice brands, including: Clausen Sweet n' Sour; Del Monte Sweet Whole Gherkins; Vlasic Bread & Butter Pickles.

REPLACEMENT: Oscar Mayer Company's Claussen Kosher Pickles

INGREDIENTS: Cucumbers, water, salt, vinegar, garlic, spices, benzoate of soda, natural flavorings, polysorbate 80.

NUTRITION PER SERVING: 1 ounce serving; 4 calories; 1 g protein; 1 g carbohydrate; less than 1 g fat; 290 mg sodium.

OTHER REPLACEMENTS: Most major brands of dill pickles.

BE ON THE LOOKOUT FOR: New Morning Naturals The Pickle Eater's Chips.

RELISH

All major brands of relish contain refined sweeteners and preservatives. Many contain artificial color as well. *Recommendation:* Use relish sparingly.

BE ON THE LOOKOUT FOR: New Morning Naturals The Pickle Eater's Relish, a no-preservative, no-refined-sugar brand from a smaller company that is beginning to be sold in supermarkets nationally.

BARBECUE SAUCE

Most major brands of bottled barbecue sauce contain sugar or corn syrup. However, as evidenced by the comparisons below, you can still make a choice that will not contain artificial ingredients or preservatives.

PRODUCT: Kraft Hickory Smoke Barbecue Sauce

INGREDIENTS: Corn syrup, tomato puree, vinegar, salt, hickory smoke flavor, modified food starch, paprika, soybean oil, molasses, spice, mustard flour, lemon juice, natural and artificial flavors, xanthan gum.

NUTRITION PER SERVING: 1 tbsp. serving; 18 calories; 1 g protein; 3 g carbohydrate; 1 g fat; 215 mg sodium.

PRODUCTS TO REPLACE: Most major brands.

REPLACEMENT: Hunt's All-Natural Thick 'n Rich Barbecue Sauce Southern Style

INGREDIENTS: Tomato concentrate, corn syrup, distilled vinegar, salt, dehydrated onions, mesquite flavor, mustard bran, spices, dehydrated carrots, garlic powder, guar gum, paprika, dehydrated celery, carob bean gum, natural flavors.

NUTRITION PER SERVING: 1 tbsp. serving; 14 calories; 1 g protein; 4 g carbohydrate; 0 g fat; 200 mg sodium.

OTHER REPLACEMENTS: Heinz 100% Natural Thick & Rich Barbecue Sauce; other Hunt's All Natural varieties.

BE ON THE LOOKOUT FOR: Enrico's Mesquite Flavor Barbecue Sauce.

Salsa

PRODUCT: La Victoria Salsa Picante

INGREDIENTS: Tomatoes, onions, jalapeños, water, tomato paste, vinegar, salt, modified food starch, sugar, coriander, garlic, benzoate of soda.

NUTRITION PER SERVING: 1 tbsp. serving; 4 calories; less than 1 g protein; 1 g carbohydrate; less than 1 g fat; 80 mg sodium.

PRODUCTS TO REPLACE: Any major brands including preservatives and sugar/corn syrup, including: Frito-Lay Chunky; Ortega Green Chili Salsa; Rosarita Chunky Salsa.

REPLACEMENT: Pace Picante Salsa Sauce

INGREDIENTS: Tomatoes, water, peppers, onions, vinegar, salt, spices.

NUTRITION PER SERVING: 2 tsp. serving; 3 calories; less than 1 g protein; less than 1 g carbohydrate; less than 1 g fat; 111 mg sodium.

OTHER REPLACEMENTS: Embassa; Old El Paso Salsa and Salsa Verde; Padrinos Hot Restaurant-Style.

SWEETENERS

PRODUCT: Sugar Twin Brown Sugar Replacement

INGREDIENTS: Dextrin, sodium saccharin, calcium chloride, caramel color, artificial flavor.

NUTRITION PER SERVING: 1 tsp. serving; less than 2 calories; 0 g protein; less than 1 g carbohydrate; 0 g fat; 0 mg sodium.

REPLACEMENT: Estee Fructose Packets

INGREDIENTS: Fructose

NUTRITION PER SERVING: 1 packet serving: 12 calories; 0 g protein; 3 g carbohydrates; 0 g fat; less than 5 mg sodium.

SPICES/SEASONINGS
(Seasoning blend; garlic salt; popcorn topping; packaged meat seasonings)

··

SEASONING BLEND

PRODUCT: Schilling Vegetable Supreme

INGREDIENTS: Salt, sesame seed, onion, monosodium glutamate, sugar, spices, natural and artificial flavorings, modified cornstarch, citric acid, disodium inosinate and guanylate, FD&C Yellow #5.

NUTRITION PER SERVING: 1 tsp. serving; 8 calories; less than 1 g protein; less than 1 g carbohydrate; less than 1 g fat; 300 mg sodium.

PRODUCTS TO REPLACE: Most major brands, including: Ac'cent Sodium-Free Herbal All-Purpose Seasoning; Morton Nature's Seasons Seasoning Blend; Schilling Salad Supreme; Schilling Salt 'n Spice.

REPLACEMENT: Salt-Free Mrs. Dash

INGREDIENTS: garlic, onion, spices (peppers, paprika, fennel, parsley, oregano, thyme, cumin, coriander, mustard, rosemary, celery seed), carrots, bell peppers, orange peel, natural flavors.

NUTRITION PER SERVING: 1 tsp. serving; 9 calories; less than 1 g protein; 2 g carbohydrate; less than 1 g fat; 0 mg sodium.

OTHER REPLACEMENTS: Chef Paul Prudhomme's Magic Seasoning blends—poultry, vegetable, seafood, meat; Health Valley All-Purpose Instead of Salt; Nu-Salt; Schilling Parsley Patch Salt-Free Lemon Pepper.

GARLIC SALT/SEASONING

PRODUCT: Schilling Garlic Salt

> **INGREDIENTS:** Salt, garlic, calcium silicate, gum arabic, garlic oil.
>
> **NUTRITION PER SERVING:** 1 tsp. serving; 3 calories; less than 1 g protein; less than 1 g carbohydrate; less than 1 g fat; 800 mg* sodium.
>
> **PRODUCTS TO REPLACE:** Most major brands, including: Schilling California-Style Blend Garlic Salt; Spice Islands Garlic Salt.

REPLACEMENT: Schilling Parsley Patch Salt-Free Garlic Saltless

> **INGREDIENTS:** Garlic, spices (including paprika), orange peel, onion, celery, red pepper.
>
> **NUTRITION PER SERVING:** ½ tsp. serving; 5 calories; less than 1 g protein; 1 g carbohydrate; 0 g fat; 1 mg sodium.

POPCORN TOPPING

PRODUCT: Molly McButter (sour cream flavor)

> **INGREDIENTS:** Maltodextrin, dehydrated buttermilk, salt, onion powder, dehydrated sour cream, dehydrated nonfat milk, natural butter flavor with other natural flavors, cornstarch, butter, lactic acid, par-

tially hydrogenated soybean oil, dehydrated parsley, tricalcium phosphate, paprika, turmeric.

NUTRITION PER SERVING: ½ tsp. serving; 4 calories; 0 g protein; 1 g carbohydrate; 0 g fat; 65 mg sodium.

REPLACEMENT: Schilling Parsley Patch Salt-Free Popcorn Blend

INGREDIENTS: Spices (including paprika), baker's yeast, onion, garlic, jalapeño pepper, lemon peel, red pepper, celery.

NUTRITION PER SERVING: ½ tsp. serving; 5 calories; .3 g protein; 1.5 g carbohydrate; 0 g fat; 2 mg sodium.

PACKAGED MEAT SEASONINGS

Many health food shoppers assume that most packaged meat seasonings (for tacos and chili) are filled with additives. Many do indeed contain sulfite agents and ingredients like silicon dioxide so that they will not cake. But there are some surprises. For instance, why not reconsider mixing your ground beef, turkey, or chicken with packaged chili seasoning rather than the taco varieties? Most of the taco varieties contain additives (including refined sugar and monosodium glutamate), while most of the chili varieties do not.

PRODUCT: Schilling Mild Taco Seasoning

INGREDIENTS: Spices (including chili pepper and paprika), onion, potato starch, salt, whey solids, monosodium glutamate, garlic, sugar, natural and artificial flavorings, citric acid.

NUTRITION PER SERVING: ⅛ package serving; 9 calories; less than 1 g protein; 3 g carbohydrates; 0 g fat; 180 mg sodium.

PRODUCTS TO REPLACE: Most major brands.

REPLACEMENT: McCormick's Chili Seasoning Mix

INGREDIENTS: Chili pepper, spices, wheat flour, onion, salt, garlic.

NUTRITION PER SERVING: ⅛ package serving; 8 calories; 0 g protein; 2 g carbohydrate; 0 g fat; 170 mg sodium.

OTHER REPLACEMENTS: Most major brands, including: Schilling.

JAM/JELLY/FRUIT SPREAD
....

PRODUCT: Smucker's   Low-Sugar   Strawberry Spread

INGREDIENTS: Strawberries, sugar, water, fruit pectin, carob bean gum, citric acid, potassium sorbate, calcium chloride, artificial colors.

NUTRITION PER SERVING: 1 tsp. serving; 8 calories; 0 g protein; 2 g carbohydrate; 0 g fat; 0 g sodium.

PRODUCTS TO REPLACE: Most other major brands, including: Kerns; Knott's Berry Farm (light or regular); Kraft preserves; Tropical; Welch's.

REPLACEMENT: Smucker's Simply Fruit Strawberry Spreadable Fruit

INGREDIENTS: White grape juice concentrate; strawberries; lemon juice concentrate; fruit pectin.

NUTRITION PER SERVING: 1 tsp. serving; 16 calories; 0 g protein; 4 g carbohydrate; 0 g fat; 0 mg sodium.

OTHER REPLACEMENTS: Smucker's Simply Fruit Spreadable Fruit flavors; Sorrell Ridge 100% Fruit flavors.

PEANUT BUTTER

PRODUCT: Jif Creamy Peanut Butter

INGREDIENTS: Peanuts, sugar, hydrogenated vegetable oil, salt, molasses, mono- and diglycerides.

NUTRITION PER SERVING: 2 tbsp. serving; 180 calories, 9 g protein; 6 g carbohydrate; 16 g fat; 155 mg sodium.

PRODUCTS TO REPLACE: Most major brands, including: Peter Pan (except version below); Skippy.

REPLACEMENT: Smucker's Natural No Salt Added Peanut Butter

INGREDIENTS: Peanuts

NUTRITION PER SERVING: 2 tbsp. serving; 200 calories; 8 g protein; 6 g carbohydrate; 17 g fat; 10 mg sodium.

OTHER REPLACEMENTS: Estee; Health Valley 100% Natural; Hollywood Natural Unsalted; Laura Scudder's Old Fashioned; Peter Pan Sodium-Free.

BUTTER/MARGARINE/ CREAMERS/COOKING OIL

BUTTER/MARGARINE

Regular margarine does not have less fat than butter. However, most have less saturated fat, although some recent studies have shown that margarine ingredients can cause your body to manufacture cholesterol. Most margarines contain preservatives and many also contain artificial ingredients, while butter is a natural food.

PRODUCT: Kraft Touch of Butter Spread

INGREDIENTS: Partially hydrogenated and liquid soybean oil, water, butter, salt, whey, sodium benzoate, lecithin, mono- and diglycerides, artificial flavor.

NUTRITION PER SERVING: 1 tbsp. serving; 90 calories; 0 g protein; 0 g carbohydrate; 10 g fat; 110 mg sodium.

PRODUCTS TO REPLACE: Most major brands, including: I Can't Believe It's Not Butter.

REPLACEMENT: Land O' Lakes Butter

INGREDIENTS: Cream, salt, annatto.

NUTRITION PER SERVING: 1 tsp. serving; 35 calories; 0 g protein; 0 g carbohydrate; 4 g fat; 40 mg sodium.

OTHER REPLACEMENTS: Most major brands, including: Challenge Butter.

PRODUCT: Imperial Stick Margarine

INGREDIENTS: Partially hydrogenated soybean and cottonseed oils, water, salt, whey, vegetable mono- and diglycerides, lecithin, sodium benzoate, artificial flavor, beta carotene, vitamin A palmitate, vitamin D calciferol.

NUTRITION PER SERVING: 1 tbsp. serving; 100 calories; 0 g protein; 0 g carbohydrates; 11 g fat; 112 mg sodium.

PRODUCTS TO REPLACE: All major brands.

REPLACEMENT: Hain Safflower Margarine

INGREDIENTS: Liquid safflower oil, partially hydrogenated soybean oil, liquid soybean oil, water, vegetable lecithin, potassium sorbate, citric acid, carotene, vitamin A palmitate.

NUTRITION PER SERVING: 1 tbsp. serving; 101 calories; less than 1 g protein; 0 g carbohydrate; 11 g fat; 6 mg sodium.

OTHER REPLACEMENTS: Hollywood Margarine.

CREAMERS

As far as nondairy creamers and cooking sprays go, you may want to switch products (as we suggest below) completely. All major brands of nondairy creamers and cooking sprays contain questionable additives.

PRODUCT: Cremora creamer

INGREDIENTS: Corn syrup solids, partially hydrogenated vegetable oils (may contain one or more of the following oils: coconut, cottonseed, palm, palm kernel; peanut or soybean), sodium casseinate (milk-derived), dipotassium phosphate, monoglycerides, sodium diacetyl, tartaric acid ester of mono- and diglycerides, artificial flavors, beta carotene, riboflavin, artificial colors.

NUTRITION PER SERVING: 1 tsp. serving; 12 calories; 0 g protein; 1 g carbohydrate; 1 g fat; 5 mg sodium.

PRODUCTS TO REPLACE: All major brands, including: Carnation Coffee-Mate.

REPLACEMENT: Any brand of nonfat milk

INGREDIENTS: Nonfat milk; vitamin A and vitamin D_3.

NUTRITION PER SERVING: ½ ounce serving; 6 calories; .6 g protein; .8 g carbohydrate; less than 1 g fat; 8 mg sodium.

OTHER REPLACEMENTS: Any brand of Half and Half.

OIL/COOKING SPRAY

PRODUCT: Mazola No Stick Corn Oil Cooking Spray

INGREDIENTS: Corn oil, lecithin, alcohol, methyl silicone, citric acid, propellant.

NUTRITION PER SERVING: .24 g serving size; 2 calories; 0 g protein; 0 g carbohydrate; less than 1 g fat, 0 mg sodium.

PRODUCTS TO REPLACE: All major brands, including: Pam.

REPLACEMENT: Wesson Corn Oil

INGREDIENTS: Corn oil

NUTRITION PER SERVING: $\frac{1}{16}$ tbsp (for pan coating) serving; 7.5 calories; 0 g protein; 0 g carbohydrate; .9 g fat; 0 mg sodium.

OTHER REPLACEMENTS: Any brand of pure vegetable (corn, peanut, sesame, canola, etc.) oil.

PRODUCT: Crisco Oil

INGREDIENTS: Vegetable oil (partially hydrogenated soybean oil), polysorbate 80, polyglycerol esters.

NUTRITION PER SERVING: 1 tbsp. serving; 120 calories; 0 g protein; 0 g carbohydrate; 14 g fat; 0 mg sodium.

REPLACEMENT: Mazola Corn Oil

INGREDIENTS: Corn oil.

NUTRITION PER SERVING: 1 tbsp. serving; 125 calories; 0 g protein; 0 g carbohydrate; 14 g fat; 0 mg sodium.

OTHER REPLACEMENTS: Any 100% vegetable oil, including: Bertolli Olive Oil; Hollywood Safflower Oil; Puritan Oil.

YOGURT

Most major brands of yogurt contain refined sugar. However, many also contain artificial ingredients and preservatives. You can skip those by making the replacement choice that follows.

PRODUCT: Knudsen Peach Lowfat Yogurt

INGREDIENTS: Cultured pasteurized milk, nonfat milk, sugar, peaches, water, modified food starch, natural flavor, Kosher gelatin, lemon juice concentrate, sodium benzoate, potassium sorbate, artificial colors.

NUTRITION PER SERVING: 1 cup serving; 240 calories; 11 g protein; 43 g carbohydrate; 4 g fat; 135 mg sodium.

PRODUCTS TO REPLACE: Most major brands, including: Other Knudsen flavors; Carnation Smooth n' Creamy flavors; Johnston's flavors; Weight Watchers flavors.

REPLACEMENT: Yoplait Original Peach Lowfat Yogurt

INGREDIENTS: Cultured pasteurized lowfat milk, nonfat milk, sugar, peaches, whey protein concentrate, natural flavors.

NUTRITION PER SERVING: 6 ounce serving; 190 calories; 8 g protein; 32 g carbohydrate; 3 g fat; 110 mg sodium.

OTHER REPLACEMENTS: Dannon flavors; other Yoplait flavors.

BE ON THE LOOKOUT FOR: Alta-Dena Nonfat Yogurts; Continental Nonfat Yogurts.

CHEESES
. . . .

A lot of cheeses are good choices because they are very natural foods. All cheeses contain enzymes used in processing, but there are many cheese products that also add lots of artificial ingredients and preservatives. The following comparisons show just how big a health difference there can be when it comes to choosing one product over another.

SWISS CHEESE

PRODUCT: Kraft Deluxe Swiss Pasteurized Process Swiss Cheese

INGREDIENTS: Swiss cheese (milk, cheese culture, salt, enzymes), water, milkfat, sodium phosphate, salt, sodium citrate, sorbic acid.

NUTRITION PER SERVING: 1 ounce serving; 90 calories; 7 g protein; 1 g carbohydrate; 7 g fat; 420 mg* sodium.

PRODUCTS TO REPLACE: Borden Lite-Line Swiss Flavor Pasteurized Process Cheese Product; Weight Watchers Swiss Flavor Pasteurized Process Cheese Product.

REPLACEMENT: Kraft Thin Deli Style Swiss Cheese Slices

INGREDIENTS: Part skim milk, cheese culture, salt, enzymes.

NUTRITION PER SERVING: 1 ounce serving; 110 calories; 8 g protein; 1 g carbohydrate; 8 g fat; 40 mg sodium.

OTHER REPLACEMENTS: Most major brands of Swiss cheese, including: Kraft Light Naturals Reduced Fat Swiss Cheese.

MONTEREY JACK

PRODUCT: Kraft Monterey Jack Pasteurized Process Cheese Singles

INGREDIENTS: Monterey cheese, water, whey, milkfat, sodium citrate, whey protein concentrate, skim milk, sodium phosphate, salt, sorbic acid.

NUTRITION PER SERVING: 1 ounce serving; 90 calories; 5 g protein; 2 g carbohydrate; 7 g fat; 390 mg sodium.

PRODUCTS TO REPLACE: Borden Lite-Line Monterey Jack Flavor Pasteurized Process Cheese Product.

REPLACEMENT: Kraft Monterey Jack Cheese Slices

INGREDIENTS: Pasteurized milk, cheese culture, salt, enzymes.

NUTRITION PER SERVING: 1 ounce serving; 110 calories; 6 g protein; 0 g carbohydrate; 9 g fat; 190 mg sodium.

OTHER REPLACEMENTS: Most brands of Monterey Jack cheese, including: Kraft Light Naturals Reduced Fat Monterey Jack Cheese Slices; Knudsen Longhorn Style Monterey Jack Cheese.

MOZZARELLA

PRODUCT: Borden Lite-Line Mozzarella Flavor Pasteurized Process Cheese Product Slices

INGREDIENTS: Skim milk cheese, low-moisture part skim mozzarella (cultured milk, skim milk, salt, enzymes), water, sodium aluminum phosphate, salt, natural flavors, sorbic acid, xanthan gum, carob bean gum, guar gum.

NUTRITION PER SERVING: ⅔ ounce serving; 35 calories; 4 g protein; 1 g carbohydrate; 2 g fat; 230 mg sodium.

REPLACEMENT: Knudsen Part-Skim Mozzarella Cheese

INGREDIENTS: Pasteurized part skim milk, cheese cultures, salt, enzymes.

NUTRITION PER SERVING: 1 ounce serving; 50 calories; 4 g protein; 1 g carbohydrate; 4 g fat; 130 mg sodium.

OTHER REPLACEMENTS: Most brands of mozzarella or part-skim mozzarella cheeses.

CREAM CHEESE

PRODUCT: Light Philadelphia Pasteurized Process Cream Cheese Product

INGREDIENTS: Cream cheese (pasteurized milk cream, cheese culture, salt, stabilizers (xanthan and/or carob bean and/or guar gums), lowfat cottage cheese (skim milk, milk, cream cheese culture, salt), skim milk, sodium citrate, lactic acid, natural flavor, vitamin A palmitate.

NUTRITION PER SERVING: 1 ounce serving; 60 calories; 3 g protein; 2 g carbohydrate; 5 g fat; 160 mg sodium.

REPLACEMENT: Philadelphia Brand Cream Cheese

INGREDIENTS: Pasteurized milk and cream, cheese culture, salt, carob bean gum.

NUTRITION PER SERVING: 1 ounce serving; 100 calories; 2 g protein; 1 g carbohydrate; 10 g fat; 85 mg sodium.

OTHER REPLACEMENTS: Most major brands of regular cream cheeses.

FLOUR/PANCAKE MIX/ SYRUP

. . . .

FLOUR

PRODUCT: Pillsbury's Best All Purpose Flour, Bleached, Enriched

INGREDIENTS: Bleached wheat flour, malted barley flour, niacin, iron, thiamine, mononitrate, riboflavin.

NUTRITION PER SERVING: 4 ounce serving: 400 calories; 11 g protein; 87 g carbohydrate; 1 g fat; 0 mg sodium.

PRODUCTS TO REPLACE: Beatrice Foods Martha White All Purpose Plain Flour, Gold Medal All Purpose Enriched Flour.

REPLACEMENT: Gold Medal Whole Wheat Flour

INGREDIENTS: Whole wheat flour, malted barley flour.

NUTRITION PER SERVING: 4 ounce serving; 390 calories; 16 g protein; 78 g carbohydrate; 2 g fat; 0 mg sodium.

OTHER REPLACEMENTS: Pillsbury's Whole Wheat Flour; Pillsbury's Best Medium Rye Flour.

PANCAKE MIX

Most major brands of pancake mix contain sugar and preservatives. Our replacement has sugar but it does not contain many of the additives of most other major brands.

PRODUCT: Aunt Jemima Pancake Mix (in shaker bottle)

INGREDIENTS: Enriched unbleached flour (flour, niacin, reduced iron, thiamine mononitrate, riboflavin), corn flour, sugar, dried buttermilk, dried whey, leavening (sodium bicarbonate, monocalcium phosphate, sodium aluminum diglycerides, salt, egg extender (soy flour, wheat flour, lecithin, partially hydrogenated cottonseed and/or soybean oil, glycerin, carrageenan), dried whole eggs, corn syrup solids, sodium caseinate.

NUTRITION PER SERVING: 3 to 4 pancake serving size: 230 calories; 7 g protein; 44 g carbohydrate; 4 g fat; 790 mg* sodium.

PRODUCTS TO REPLACE: Most major brands, including: Aunt Jemima Complete Buttermilk Pancake Mix; Betty Crocker Complete Buttermilk Pancake Mix; Bisquick Shake 'n Pour; Pillsbury Hungry Jack.

REPLACEMENT: Hungry Jack Buttermilk Pancake and Waffle Mix

INGREDIENTS: Enriched flour (flour, niacin, iron, thiamine mononitrate, riboflavin), sugar, rice flour, baking powder (baking soda, sodium aluminum phosphate), buttermilk, salt.

NUTRITION PER SERVING: 3 pancake serving; 240 calories; 7 g protein; 29 g carbohydrate; 11 g fat; 570 mg* sodium.

BE ON THE LOOKOUT FOR: David's Goodbatter Pancake and Baking Mix.

SYRUP

PRODUCT: Aunt Jemima Syrup Extra Thick

INGREDIENTS: Corn syrup, water, cellulose gum, natural and artificial flavors, salt, sodium benzoate, sorbic acid, caramel color.

NUTRITION PER SERVING: 1 fluid ounce serving; 109 calories; 0 g protein; 27.19 g carbohydrate; 0 g fat; 32 mg sodium.

PRODUCTS TO REPLACE: Most major brands, including: Golden Griddle; Kellogg's Eggo; Knott's Berry Farm Natural Syrups; Log Cabin; Smucker's Natural Syrups.

REPLACEMENT: MacDonald's Premium Maple Syrup

INGREDIENTS: Maple syrup

NUTRITION PER SERVING: 1 tbsp. serving; 50 calories; 0 g protein; 13 g carbohydrate; less than 1 g fat; 4 mg sodium.

OTHER REPLACEMENTS: All other maple syrups, including: Camp 100% Pure Maple Syrup; Cary's Maple Syrup; Reese Pure Maple Syrup.

CANNED FRUIT/ APPLE SAUCE/ CANNED VEGETABLES/ FROZEN VEGETABLES AND PACKAGED VEGETABLES

. . . .

CANNED FRUIT

PRODUCT: Del Monte Sliced Cling Peaches in Heavy Syrup

INGREDIENTS: Peaches, water, corn syrup, sugar.

NUTRITION PER SERVING: ½ cup serving; 80 calories; 0 g protein; 22 g carbohydrate; 0 g fat; 110 mg sodium.

PRODUCTS TO REPLACE: All brands with sugar or artificial sweeteners, including: Del Monte Lite Apricot halves; Del Monte Lite Fruit Cocktail; Del Monte Light

Pear Halves; Del Monte Pear Halves in Heavy Syrup; Dole Mandarin Orange Slices; Dole Pineapple Chunks in Heavy Syrup; Dole Pineapple Slices in Heavy Syrup.

REPLACEMENT: Del Monte Fruit Naturals, Sliced Peaches

INGREDIENTS: Peaches, peach juice

NUTRITION PER SERVING: ½ cup serving; 60 calories; 0 g protein; 15 g carbohydrate; 0 g fat; 10 mg sodium.

OTHER REPLACEMENTS: Del Monte Fruit Naturals Pear Halves; Dole Crushed Pineapple in Unsweetened Pineapple Juice; Dole Pineapple Chunks in Unsweetened Pineapple Juice; Libby's Lite Sliced Peaches; Libby's Lite Sliced Pears; S & W Natural-Style Mandarin Orange Slices; S & W Sliced Quartered Pears; S & W Sliced Peaches; Springfield Sliced Cling Peaches in Pear Juice.

APPLE SAUCE

PRODUCT: Original Tree Top Apple Sauce

INGREDIENTS: Apples, corn syrup, sugar, water, ascorbic acid.

NUTRITION PER SERVING: ½ cup serving; 80 calories; 0 g protein; 21 g carbohydrate; 0 g fat; 0 g sodium.

PRODUCTS TO REPLACE: Apple Time Apple Sauce; Apple Time Cinnamon Apple Sauce; Mott's Apple Sauce; Mott's Chunky Apple Sauce; Seneca Spoonpak Cinnamon Apple Sauce.

REPLACEMENT: Mott's Natural Apple Sauce

INGREDIENTS: Apples, water.

NUTRITION PER SERVING: 4 fluid ounce serving; 53 calories; 0 g protein; 13 g carbohydrate; 0 g fat; 2 mg sodium.

OTHER REPLACEMENTS: Apple Time Original Apple Sauce with Cinnamon; Apple Time Original Unsweetened Apple Sauce; Musselman Unsweetened Apple Sauce; S & W Unsweetened Apple Sauce; Seneca 100% Natural Apple Sauce; Seneca Spoonpak Apple Sauce.

CANNED VEGETABLE

Most canned and frozen/packaged vegetable products are just vegetables. You'll find a lot of good choices. However, there are some major brands that hide sugar and other additives in their products.

PRODUCT: Green Giant Niblets Golden Sweet Corn

INGREDIENTS: Corn, water, sugar, salt.

NUTRITION PER SERVING: ½ cup serving; 80 calories; 2 g protein; 20 g carbohydrate; 0 g fat; 330 mg* sodium.

PRODUCTS TO REPLACE: All brands containing sugar, including: Del Monte Creamed Style Golden Sweet Corn; Green Giant Mexicorn; Green Giant White Corn; S & W Whole Kernel Corn; Veg-all Freshlike Mixed Vegetables.

REPLACEMENT: Del Monte Whole Kernel Corn

INGREDIENTS: Corn, water, salt.

NUTRITION PER SERVING: ½ cup serving; 45 calories; 2 g protein; 10 g carbohydrate; 0 g fat; 369 mg sodium.

OTHER REPLACEMENTS: All brands that contain no sugar, including Libby's Natural Packaged Mixed Vegetables, Veg-All Freshlike Lite Mixed Vegetables.

PACKAGED OR FROZEN VEGETABLES

PRODUCT: Del Monte Vegetable Classics Tiny Sweet Peas and Sliced Mushrooms (packaged product usually stocked near canned vegetables)

INGREDIENTS: Peas, water, mushrooms, margarine (corn oil, partially hydrogenated corn oil, water, salt, whey, mono- and diglycerides, lecithin, artificial flavors and colors, vitamin A palmitate, vitamin D, modified food starch, salt, sugar, natural flavors, guar gum, hydroxylated lecithin, spice, xanthan gum, FD&C Yellow No. 5.

NUTRITION PER SERVING: ½ cup serving; 70 calories; 3 g protein; 9 g carbohydrate; 2 g fat; 430 mg* sodium.

REPLACEMENT: Green Giant Frozen Sweet Peas

INGREDIENTS: Sweet peas, salt.

NUTRITION PER SERVING: ½ cup serving; 60 calories; 4 g protein; 11 g carbohydrate; 0 g fat; 110 mg sodium.

OTHER REPLACEMENTS: All brands that contain no sugar, preservatives, and artificial ingredients.

PRODUCT: Del Monte Vegetable Classics Sweet Corn and Julienne Carrots (packaged and usually stocked near canned vegetables)

INGREDIENTS: Corn, carrots, water, margarine (corn oil, partially hydrogenated corn oil, water, salt, whey, mono- and diglycerides, lecithin, artificial flavor and color, vitamin A palmitate, vitamin D), modified food starch, salt, natural flavors, guar gum, spices, citric acid, xanthan gum, color.

NUTRITION PER SERVING: ½ cup serving; 70 calories; 1 g protein; 12 g carbohydrate; 2 g fat; 310 mg sodium.

REPLACEMENT: Birds Eye Farm Fresh Mixtures Broccoli, Corn and Red Peppers

INGREDIENTS: Broccoli, corn, red peppers.

NUTRITION PER SERVING: ½ cup serving; 60 calories; 3 g protein; 14 g carbohydrate; 1 g fat; 15 mg sodium.

OTHER REPLACEMENTS: All packaged or frozen vegetables that contain no sugar, preservatives, and artificial ingredients.

SOUP/CANNED CHILI/ CANNED MAIN DISHES/ CANNED TUNA

SOUP: CHICKEN BROTH

PRODUCT: Campbell's Chicken Broth

INGREDIENTS: Chicken broth, chicken fat, salt, yeast extract and hydrolyzed vegetable protein, monosodium glutamate, dextrose and natural flavoring.

NUTRITION PER SERVING: 4 ounce serving; 35 calories; 1 g protein; 3 g carbohydrate; 2 g fat; 750 mg* sodium.

PRODUCTS TO REPLACE: Most other major brands, including: Swanson Chicken Broth.

REPLACEMENT: Pritikin Chicken Broth

INGREDIENTS: Chicken broth, carrots, natural flavor.

NUTRITION PER SERVING: 6.2 ounce serving; 12 calories; 2 g protein; 1 g carbohydrate; 0 g fat; 135 mg sodium.

OTHER REPLACEMENTS: Health Valley.

SOUP: MUSHROOM/VEGETABLE/LENTIL

PRODUCT: Campbell's Cream of Mushroom Soup

INGREDIENTS: Water, mushrooms, vegetable oil (corn, cottonseed or partially hydrogenated soybean oil), wheat flour, cream, salt, cornstarch, dried dairy blend (whey, calcium casseinate), modified food starch, whey, monosodium glutamate, soy protein isolate), natural flavoring, yeast extract, dehydrated garlic.

NUTRITION PER SERVING: 4 ounce serving; 100 calories; 2 g protein; 8 g carbohydrate; 7 g fat; 820 mg* sodium.

PRODUCTS TO REPLACE: Most major brands, including: Campbell's Chicken Vegetable Soup; Campbell's Home Cookin' Country Vegetable; Campbell's Home Cookin' Lentil; Campbell's Home Cookin' Vegetable Beef; Campbell's Special Request Vegetable Beef; Pepperidge Farms Shiitake Mushroom Soup; Progresso Home Style Chicken with Vegetables.

REPLACEMENT: Campbell's Natural Creamy Broccoli Soup

INGREDIENTS: Chicken stock, broccoli, cream, wheat flour, water, butter, eggs, salt, cornstarch, dehydrated onions, natural flavoring.

NUTRITION PER SERVING: 1 cup serving; 140 calories; 5 g protein; 13 g carbohydrate; 8 g fat; 875 mg* sodium.

OTHER REPLACEMENTS: Campbell's Natural Creamy Potato Soup; Hain Naturals Lentil Soup Hearty Home Style; Hain Naturals Mushroom Soup; Hain Vegetarian Vegetable Soup; Health Valley Natural Lentil Soup; Health Valley Natural Vegetable Soup; Progresso Lentil Soup; Tabatchnick Soups (freezer section).

SOUP: DRIED SOUP

All major brands of dried soups contain refined sweeteners and preservatives and/or artificial ingredients. Recommendation: If possible, stick to liquid soups that contain no sugar or other additives.

BE ON THE LOOKOUT FOR: The Spice Hunter Quick and Natural Soups and Just Delicious Soup Mixes. These are brands from smaller companies that have no sugar, preservatives, or additives. They are being introduced in supermarkets nationally.

CANNED CHILI/BEANS

Most canned chili products contain sugar and additives such as modified food starch, but most canned refried bean entrées do not. After seeing our comparison, you might want to think about serving refried beans. You'll also be serving your family fewer calories, a lot less fat, and somewhat less sodium.

PRODUCT: Hormel Chili with Beans

INGREDIENTS: Water, beef, beans, tomatoes, chili powder (chili peppers, flavoring), corn flour, salt, modified food starch, sugar, flavoring.

NUTRITION PER SERVING: 7.5 ounce serving size; 250 calories; 15 g protein; 23 g carbohydrate; 11 g fat; 980 mg* sodium.

PRODUCTS TO REPLACE: Most major brands, including: Dennison's Chunky Chili Con Carne with Beans; Dennison's Lite Chili with Beans; Stagg Country Chili; Stagg Steak House Chili without Beans.

REPLACEMENT: Old El Paso Refried Beans

INGREDIENTS: Cooked beans, water, salt, lard.

NUTRITION PER SERVING: 1 cup serving, 200 calories; 14 g protein; 34 g carbohydrate; 2 g fat; 600 mg* sodium.

OTHER REPLACEMENTS: Most major brands.

BE ON THE LOOKOUT FOR: Health Valley Mild Vegetarian Chili with Beans or Lentils.

CANNED MAIN DISHES: ITALIAN FOOD

Most canned main dish entrées contain corn syrup or other sweeteners. However, if you're going to partake, leaving monosodium glutamate and a processed coloring off your family's dinner plates is as easy as picking Chef Boyardee Lasagna over Chef Boyardee Beef Ravioli.

PRODUCT: Chef Boyardee Beef Ravioli

INGREDIENTS: Tomatoes, water, enriched wheat flour, beef, cracker meal, salt, carrots, high fructose corn syrup, modified food starch, rendered beef fat, textured vegetable protein (soy flour, caramel coloring), caramel coloring, monosodium glutamate, onions, flavorings, enzyme modified cheese.

NUTRITION PER SERVING: 8 ounce serving; 220 calories; 8 g protein; 35 g carbohydrate; 5 g fat; 1120 mg* sodium.

PRODUCTS TO REPLACE: Most major brands.

REPLACEMENT: Chef Boyardee Lasagna

INGREDIENTS: Tomatoes, water, beef, enriched lasagna macaroni product, high fructose corn syrup, salt, modified food starch, enzyme modified cheese, onions, flavorings.

NUTRITION PER SERVING: 7.5 ounce serving; 220 calories; 8 g protein; 28 g carbohydrates; 9 g fat; 1,000 mg* sodium.

CANNED MAIN DISHES: TAMALES

PRODUCT: Old El Paso Tamales in Chili Sauce

INGREDIENTS: Water, corn flour, beef, pork, chili powder, wheat flour, tomato paste, salt, oatmeal flakes, cumin, sugar, red pepper powder, oregano, onion powder, garlic powder, sage.

NUTRITION PER SERVING: 2 tamale serving; 232 calories; 6 g protein; 23 g carbohydrate; 13 g* fat; 700 mg* sodium.

REPLACEMENT: Hormel Beef Tamales in Chili Sauce

INGREDIENTS: Water, beef, tomatoes, corn meal, corn flour, masa harina, salt, chili powder (chili peppers, natural flavorings), paprika, spice.

NUTRITION PER SERVING: 2 tamale serving; 140 calories; 4 g protein; 8 g carbohydrate; 10 g fat; 550 mg* sodium.

OTHER REPLACEMENTS: Nalley Beef Canned Tamales.

CANNED MAIN DISHES: BEEF STEW

PRODUCT: Dinty Moore Beef Stew

INGREDIENTS: Beef broth, beef, potatoes, carrots, corn flour, beef fat, salt, tomato paste, modified food starch, sugar, caramel coloring, flavoring.

NUTRITION PER SERVING: 7.5 ounce serving; 180 calories; 12 g protein; 14 g carbohydrate; 9 g fat; 939 mg* sodium.

PRODUCTS TO REPLACE: Most major brands.

REPLACEMENT: Featherweight Beef Stew with Vegetables

INGREDIENTS: Beef broth (natural flavor, salt), cooked beef, water, dehydrated potatoes, carrots, corn, peas, celery, modified food starch, green beans, wheat flour, tomato paste, burgundy wine, dehydrated bell peppers, natural flavor, salt, paprika.

NUTRITION PER SERVING: 7.5 ounce serving; 160 calories; 17 g protein; 17 g carbohydrate; 3 g fat; 400 mg sodium.

CANNED MAIN DISH: CHICKEN PRODUCTS

PRODUCT: Libby's Spreadables Ready to Serve Chicken Salad

INGREDIENTS: Cooked chicken, water, vegetable oil (soybean and/or cottonseed), vinegar, sugar, water chestnuts, pickles, textured soy flour, modified food starch, cellulose gel and gum, salt, titanium dioxide, flavorings, polysorbate 60, monosodium glutamate, turmeric.

NUTRITION PER SERVING: ¼ can serving; 100 calories; 6 g protein; 7 g carbohydrate; 7 g fat; 220 mg sodium.

PRODUCTS TO REPLACE: Most major brands.

REPLACEMENT: Swanson Premium Chunk White Chicken in Water

INGREDIENTS: Chicken breast meat, water, salt, natural flavoring.

NUTRITION PER SERVING: 2.5 ounce serving; 80 calories; 16 g protein; 1 g carbohydrate; 2 g fat; 250 mg sodium.

OTHER REPLACEMENTS: Hormel Chunk Breast of Chicken; Valley Fresh Premium Chunk White Chicken in Broth.

CANNED TUNA

PRODUCT: Star-Kist Solid White Tuna in Water

INGREDIENTS: White tuna, water, vegetable broth, salt, pyrophosphate.

NUTRITION PER SERVING: ½ cup serving; 110 calories; 23 g protein; 0 g carbohydrate; 2 g fat; 350 mg sodium.

PRODUCTS TO REPLACE: Chicken of the Sea Solid White Tuna in Oil, Chicken of the Sea Chunk Light Tuna in Water.

REPLACEMENT: Bumble Bee Chunk Light Tuna in Water

INGREDIENTS: Chunk light tuna in water, salt.

NUTRITION PER SERVING: ½ cup serving; 117 calories; 26 g protein; 0 g carbohydrates; 1 g fat; 311 mg sodium.

OTHER REPLACEMENTS: Most major brands that are packed in water.

RICE/RICE MIXES

RICE

PRODUCT: MJB Quick Enriched Brown Rice

INGREDIENTS: Brown rice, thiamine, riboflavin, iron, BHT, cottonseed oil, cellulose gum.

NUTRITION PER SERVING: ½ cup serving size; 110 calories; 2 g protein; 22 g carbohydrate; 1 g fat; 0 g sodium.

PRODUCTS TO REPLACE: Most other major brands, including: Original Minute Rice (Enriched); Uncle Ben's Aromatic Natural Long-Grain Rice; Uncle Ben's Converted Enriched Rice.

REPLACEMENT: Minute Brand Instant Brown Rice

INGREDIENTS: Precooked long grain brown rice.

NUTRITION PER SERVING: 1.1 ounce serving; 120 calories; 3 g protein; 26 g carbohydrate; 1 g fat; 5 mg sodium.

OTHER REPLACEMENTS: Most other brown rices, including: Success Brown Rice; Uncle Ben's Whole Grain Brown Rice.

RICE MIXES: PILAF

PRODUCT: Rice-A-Roni Rice Pilaf

INGREDIENTS: Enriched parboiled long grain rice, enriched macaroni product, salt, natural flavors, modified food starch, chicken fat, dried yeast, monosodium glutamate, dried onions, dried chicken broth, spice, dried garlic, dried chives, disodium guanylate, turmeric extract, BHA, propyl gallate.

NUTRITION PER SERVING: 1.2 ounce (dry mix) serving size; 120 calories; 4 g protein; 25 g carbohydrate; 1 g fat; 570 mg* sodium.

PRODUCTS TO REPLACE: Most other major brands, including: MJB Rice Pilaf.

REPLACEMENT: Near East Rice Pilaf Mix

INGREDIENTS: Parboiled long grain rice, orzo macaroni product (semolina), salt, natural flavors, turmeric, onion powder, garlic powder.

NUTRITION PER SERVING: ½ cup serving (dry mix); 100 calories; 3 g protein; 22 g carbohydrate; 1 g fat; 400 mg* sodium.

OTHER REPLACEMENTS: Near East Barley Pilaf; Near East Beef Flavor Rice Pilaf.

BE ON THE LOOKOUT FOR: Casbah pilafs.

RICE MIXES: CHICKEN FLAVOR (AND OTHER SIDE DISHES)

PRODUCT: Rice-A-Roni Chicken Flavor

INGREDIENTS: Enriched rice, enriched vermicelli, salt, modified food starch, natural flavors, sugar, chicken fat, dehydrated onions, monosodium glutamate, dehydrated chicken broth, dehydrated chicken, dehydrated parsley, dehydrated yeast, soy flour, dehydrated garlic, spices, partially hydrogenated vegetable oil (soybean and/or cottonseed), disodium guanylate, BHA, propyl gallate.

NUTRITION PER SERVING: 1.13 ounce (32 g) dry mix serving; 110 calories; 3 g protein; 24 g carbohydrate; 1 g fat, 520 mg* sodium.

PRODUCTS TO REPLACE: Most major brands, including: Lipton Rice and Sauce Creamy Chicken flavor; MJB Savory Chicken flavor; Rice-A-Roni Savory Classics Chicken flavor; Uncle Ben's Country Inn Homestyle Chicken and Vegetables flavor.

Almost all packaged rice products contain sugar, monosodium glutamate, and a lot of other additives. Following are some of the few that are widely available that contain none of those additives.

REPLACEMENT: Pritikin Spanish Brown Rice

INGREDIENTS: Precooked long grain brown rice, tomato powder, dried onion, green pepper flakes, garlic powder, dried parsley flakes, rice flour, spice, cornstarch.

NUTRITION PER SERVING: ½ cup serving; 100 calories; 3 g protein; 21 g carbohydrate; less than 1 g fat; 15 mg sodium.

OTHER REPLACEMENTS: Hain Rice Almondine; Hain Rice Oriental; Hain 3 Grain Chicken Side Dish; Hain 3 Grain Herb; Near East Spanish Rice Mix.

SPAGHETTI (PASTA)/ MACARONI AND CHEESE MIX/SPAGHETTI SAUCE/ PIZZA SAUCE/TOMATO SAUCE

SPAGHETTI (PASTA)

Spaghetti and pasta are excellent complex carbohydrates. But the goal here, as described in the text of the book, is if possible to avoid enriched products. Many pasta products are enriched.

PRODUCT: Creamette Brand Thin Spaghetti

INGREDIENTS: Semolina, enriched with niacinamide, ferrous sulfate, thiamine mononitrate, riboflavin.

NUTRITION PER SERVING: 2 ounce (dry) serving; 210 calories; 7 g protein; 42 g carbohydrate; 1 g fat; 2 mg sodium.

PRODUCTS TO REPLACE: Most major brands, including: American Beauty; Anthony's Macaroni Products; Prince Enriched Macaroni, Spaghetti and Superoni.

REPLACEMENT: Ronzoni Spaghetti

INGREDIENTS: Durum wheat, No. 1 semolina

NUTRITION PER SERVING: 2 ounce (dry) serving; 210 calories; 7 g protein; 41 g carbohydrates; 1 g fat; less than 5 mg sodium.

OTHER REPLACEMENTS: De Bole Thin Spaghetti or Whole Wheat Spaghetti and pasta products; Health Valley Organic Spinach Spaghetti Pasta; Health Valley Whole Wheat Lasagna with wheat germ; Pritikin Whole Wheat Ribbon Pasta; Pritikin Whole Wheat Spaghetti.

MACARONI AND CHEESE MIX

PRODUCT: Kraft Macaroni and Cheese Dinner

INGREDIENTS: Enriched macaroni, cheese sauce mix (whey, dehydrated cheese—granular and cheddar [milk, cheese culture, salt, enzymes]), whey protein concentrate, skim milk, salt, buttermilk, sodium tripolyphosphate, sodium phosphate, citric acid, Yellow No. 5 & 6, lactic acid.

NUTRITION PER SERVING: ¾ cup prepared serving; 290 calories; 9 g protein; 34 g carbohydrate; 13 g* fat; 530 mg* salt.

PRODUCTS TO REPLACE: Most major brands, including: Creamettes Macaroni and Cheese; Golden Grain Macaroni and Cheddar; Minute Microwave Pasta and Cheddar Cheese; Springfield Enriched Macaroni and Cheese Dinner; Velveeta Shells and Cheese.

REPLACEMENT: De Bole's Whole Wheat Macaroni

INGREDIENTS: Organically grown durum whole wheat flour, cheese (corn flour, cheddar cheese, buttermilk, natural cheese flavor).

NUTRITION PER SERVING: 2 ounce serving; 200 calories; 8 g protein; 39 g carbohydrate; 2 g fat; 225 mg sodium.

OTHER REPLACEMENTS: De Bole's Macaroni and Cheese Dinner; Hain Creamy Parmesan Pasta and Sauce; Hain Fettucine Alfredo; Hain Tangy Cheddar Pasta and Sauce.

SPAGHETTI SAUCE

PRODUCT: Ragú Old World Style 100% Natural Spaghetti Sauce with Meat

INGREDIENTS: Tomatoes (water, tomato paste), soybean oil, beef, salt, sugar, corn syrup, dried onions, olive oil, spices, Romano cheese made from cow's milk, natural garlic flavor.

NUTRITION PER SERVING: 4 ounce serving size; 80 calories; 2 g protein; 11 g carbohydrate; 2 g fat; 740 mg* sodium.

PRODUCTS TO REPLACE: Most major brands that include refined sweeteners, including: Hunt's brands (except Homestyle Traditional); Newman's Own brands; Prego brands (except no-sugar-added brand); additional Ragú brands (except no-sugar-added version).

REPLACEMENT: Ragú (No Sugar Added) Homestyle 100% Natural Spaghetti Sauce

INGREDIENTS: Tomatoes (water, tomato paste), soybean oil, salt, dried onions, parsley, olive oil, basil, oregano, black pepper, thyme, natural garlic flavor.

NUTRITION PER SERVING: 4 ounce serving size; 70 calories; 2 g protein; 11 g carbohydrate; 2 g fat; 390 mg sodium.

OTHER REPLACEMENTS: Classico Tomato and Basil Pasta Sauce; Classico Spicy Red Pepper Pasta Sauce; Hunt's Homestyle Traditional Spaghetti Sauce (no sugar added); Hunt's Homestyle with Mushrooms (no sugar added); Prego (no salt added, no sugar added) Spaghetti Sauce; Aunt Millie's Meatless Traditional Spaghetti Sauce or Spaghetti Sauce with Sweet Peppers and Italian Sausage (made by Prince Macaroni); Progresso Marinara Spaghetti Sauce with Mushrooms; Sinatra's Milano-style Marinara Sauce.

PIZZA SAUCE

PRODUCT: Ragú Pizza Quick Sauce Traditional

INGREDIENTS: Tomatoes (water, tomato paste), soybean oil, salt, modified food starch, dried onions, sugar, spices, corn syrup, natural garlic flavor.

NUTRITION PER SERVING: 3 tbsp. serving size; 40 calories; 1 g protein; 4 g carbohydrate; 2 g fat; 300 mg sodium.

PRODUCTS TO REPLACE: Most major brands, including: Contadina.

REPLACEMENT: Ragú 100% Natural Pizza Sauce

INGREDIENTS: Tomatoes (water, tomato paste), soybean oil, salt, spices, parsley, natural garlic flavor.

NUTRITION PER SERVING: 3 tbsp. serving; 25 calories; 1 g protein; 3 g carbohydrate, 1 g fat, 200 mg sodium.

BE ON THE LOOKOUT FOR: Enrico's Pizza Sauce.

TOMATO SAUCE

PRODUCT: Del Monte Tomato Sauce

INGREDIENTS: Tomatoes, salt, pepper, corn sweetener, spice.

NUTRITION PER SERVING: ½ cup serving; 35 calories; 2 g protein; 8 g carbohydrate; less than 1 g fat; 665 mg* sodium.

PRODUCTS TO REPLACE: All major brands containing refined sweeteners or additives, including: Hunt's.

REPLACEMENT: Contadina Tomato Sauce

INGREDIENTS: Tomatoes, salt, spices, garlic powder.

NUTRITION PER SERVING: ½ cup serving; 45 calories; 2 g protein; 9 g carbohydrate; 0 g fat; 510 mg* sodium.

OTHER REPLACEMENTS: All brands containing no refined sweeteners or additives.

FRANKFURTERS/COLD CUTS/BACON/SAUSAGE

FRANKFURTERS

All major brands of frankfurters, whether beef, pork, chicken or turkey, contain nitrites, which have been shown to have possible links to cancer. They also contain other curing agents. However, hot dogs are an all-American food, and if we're going to eat them, some brands stand above the rest because they contain no sugar. We'll look at both "light" and regular franks.

PRODUCT: Oscar Mayer Light Beef Franks

INGREDIENTS: Beef, water, salt, corn syrup, dextrose (also corn syrup), hydrolyzed milk protein, flavoring, sodium phosphates, sodium erythorbate, extractives of paprika, sodium nitrite.

NUTRITION PER SERVING: 1 frank serving; 130 calories; 7 g protein; 1 g carbohydrate; 11 g fat; 600 mg* sodium.

PRODUCTS TO REPLACE: All major brands, including beef, pork, chicken, and turkey.

REPLACEMENT: Ballpark Lite Franks

INGREDIENTS: Pork, water, turkey meat, beef, salt, flavoring, sodium erythorbate, sodium nitrite, oleoresin paprika.

NUTRITION PER SERVING: 1 frank serving; 140 calories; 7 g protein; 1 g carbohydrate; 11 g fat; 390 mg sodium.

BE ON THE LOOKOUT FOR: The following brands have no nitrites, preservatives, or refined sweeteners: Health Valley Naturally Spiced Uncured Turkey Wieners; Shelton's brands of chicken or turkey franks.

PRODUCT: Oscar Mayer Bun-Length Wieners

INGREDIENTS: Pork, water, beef, salt, corn syrup, dextrose (also corn syrup), flavoring, sodium erythorbate, oleoresin paprika, sodium nitrite.

NUTRITION PER SERVING: 1 wiener serving; 180 calories; 6 g protein; 2 g carbohydrate; 17 g* fat; 590 mg* sodium.

PRODUCTS TO REPLACE: All major brands.

REPLACEMENT: Hebrew National Beef Franks

INGREDIENTS: Beef, water, salt, spice, paprika, hydrolized vegetable protein, garlic powder, sodium erythorbate, sodium nitrite, natural flavorings.

NUTRITION PER SERVING: 1 frank serving: 140 calories; 6 g protein; 3 g carbohydrate; 14 g* fat; 480 mg* sodium.

OTHER REPLACEMENTS: Ballpark Beef Franks; Nathan's Beef Franks.

COLD CUTS

Almost all major brands of cold cuts contain nitrites, a controversial additive that has been shown to cause cancer in laboratory animals, as well as preservatives. However, many cold cuts also contain refined sweeteners. A few, though, stand out because they do not contain refined sweeteners, as the following comparisons show. Recommendation: Eat packaged cold cuts sparingly, and buy cold cuts, if possible, in your supermarket's fresh deli section, where supermarket clerks will cut the meat for you. These meats will have fewer preservatives and you can ask for those that do not contain sugar.

PRODUCT: Louis Rich Oven Roasted Turkey Breast

INGREDIENTS: Turkey breast, turkey broth, sodium lactate, modified food starch, salt, sugar, sodium phosphates.

NUTRITION PER SERVING: 1 slice serving; 30 calories; 5 g protein; 1 g carbohydrate; less than 1 g fat; 340 mg sodium.

PRODUCTS TO REPLACE: All major brands, including: Armour; Buddig; Hillshire Farms; Oscar Mayer.

REPLACEMENT: Swift-Eckrich's Butterball Turkey Breast Oven Roasted

INGREDIENTS: Turkey breast, water, sodium lactate, modified food starch, salt, sodium phosphates, flavoring.

NUTRITION PER SERVING: 1 slice serving; 30 calories; 5 g protein; 1 g carbohydrate; 1 g fat; 280 mg sodium.

PRODUCT: Oscar Mayer Thin Sliced Roast Chicken Breast

INGREDIENTS: Chicken breast, water, sodium lactate, dextrose (corn syrup), salt, carageenan, sodium phosphates.

NUTRITION PER SERVING: 2 slice serving; 28 calories; 4 g protein; 2 g carbohydrate; 2 g fat; 320 mg sodium.

REPLACEMENT: Louis Rich Oven Roasted White Chicken

INGREDIENTS: White chicken, chicken broth, nonfat dry milk, sodium lactate, salt, carageenan, sodium phosphates.

NUTRITION PER SERVING: 1 slice serving (thicker than Oscar Mayer above); 35 calories; 5 g protein; less than 1 g carbohydrate; 2 g fat; 310 mg sodium.

BACON

All major brands of bacon contain nitrites and refined sugar. *Recommendation:* Eat bacon sparingly.

SAUSAGE

PRODUCT: Swift Original Brown 'n Serve Beef Links

INGREDIENTS: Beef, water, salt, sugar, spices, monosodium glutamate, BHA, BHT, citric acid.

NUTRITION PER SERVING: 1 link serving; 221 calories; 13 g protein; less than 1 g carbohydrate; 18 g* fat; 850 mg* sodium.

PRODUCTS TO REPLACE: All major brands.

REPLACEMENT: Jones Little Sausages

INGREDIENTS: Pork, salt, spices

NUTRITION PER SERVING: 1 link serving; 200 calories; 12 g protein; less than 1 g carbohydrate; 16 g* fat; 539 mg* sodium.

BE ON THE LOOKOUT FOR: Shelton's Turkey Breakfast Sausage, which has no sweeteners or preservatives.

FROZEN FOODS

. . . .

FISH

PRODUCT: Gorton's Light Recipe Baked Stuffed Scrod

INGREDIENTS: Haddock, butter, bromated wheat flour, lemon juice, water, salt, parsley, sugar, partially dehydrated soybean oil with TBHQ, yeast, calcium propionate.

NUTRITION PER SERVING: 240 calories; 25 g protein; 11 g carbohydrate; 11 g* fat; 470 mg* sodium.

PRODUCTS TO REPLACE: Gorton's Light Recipe Fish Fillets; Mrs. Paul's Crispy Crunchy Fish Sticks; Taste O'Sea Batter Dipt Scallops.

REPLACEMENT: Gorton's Fishmarket Fresh Ocean Perch Fillets

INGREDIENTS: Ocean perch fillets.

NUTRITION PER SERVING: 4 ounce serving; 130 calories; 20 g protein; 2 g carbohydrate; 5 g fat; 80 mg sodium.

PRODUCT: Mrs. Paul's Light and Natural Sole Fillets

INGREDIENTS: Sole fillets, bread crumbs (bromated wheat flour, sugar, partially hydrogenated soybean oil, salt, yeast, calcium propionate), enriched flour (flour, niacin, reduced iron, thiamine mononitrate or thiamine hydrochloride, riboflavin), partially hydrogenated soybean oil, corn flour, whey, modified food starch, dextrose, salt, whole egg solids, sodium aluminum phosphate, sodium bicarbonate, wheat gluten.

NUTRITION PER SERVING: 1 fillet serving; 280 calories; 21 g protein; 19 g carbohydrate; 13 g* fat; 390 mg sodium.

REPLACEMENT: Gorton's Fishmarket Fresh Sole Fillets

INGREDIENTS: Sole fillets.

NUTRITION PER SERVING: 4 ounce serving; 100 calories; 19 g protein; 0 g carbohydrate; 3 g fat; 260 mg sodium.

FROZEN DINNERS

Almost all major brands of packaged frozen dinners—whether regular or "light" or "healthy"—contain refined sweeteners and many other additives. However, there are some with no sugar and many fewer additives and artificial ingredients. The comparisons that follow show that there can be huge health differences when it comes to products that are seemingly similar. For instance, the first comparison shows you can still choose a Hungry-Man entrée, and yet cut way down on calories, fat, and sodium.

PRODUCT: Swanson Hungry-Man Chopped Beef Steak Dinner

INGREDIENTS: Chopped beef steak (beef, reconstituted onions, salt, spice, natural flavoring), reconstituted dehydrated potatoes, beef stock, green beans, water, graham cracker crumbs (graham cracker meal [enriched flour, wheat flour, graham flour, sugar, partially hydrogenated vegetable oil, corn syrup, brown sugar, salt, malt, baking soda], brown sugar, vegetable shortening, natural flavoring), dehydrated apples, margarine, black raspberries, blueberries, modified food starch, sugar, sherry wine, salt, vegetable oil, wheat flour, tomato paste, dried whey, onion powder, butter, dry garlic, caramel color, natural flavoring, spice.

NUTRITION PER SERVING: 17.25 ounce serving; 620 calories; 30 g protein; 42 g carbohydrate; 37 g* fat; 2,030 mg* sodium.

PRODUCTS TO REPLACE: Most major brands, including: Armour; Banquet; Lean Cuisine; Morton; Stouffer's; Swanson; Weight Watchers.

REPLACEMENT: Swanson Hungry-Man Sliced Beef

INGREDIENTS: Cooked beef, reconstituted dehydrated potatoes, beef stock, water, margarine, modified food starch, salt, tomato paste, wheat flour, dried whey, yeast extract, hydrolyzed plant protein, onion powder, monosodium glutamate, butter, caramel color, natural flavoring, dehydrated garlic.

NUTRITION PER SERVING: 12.25 ounce serving; 330 calories; 40 g protein; 24 g carbohydrate; 8 g fat; 1,045 mg* sodium.

OTHER REPLACEMENTS: Banquet Buffet Supper Gravy and Sliced Beef; Le Menu Beef Sirloin Tips Dinner or Breast of Chicken Dinner; Morton Sloppy Joe

Frozen Boil-in-the-Bag Entrée; Weaver Good 'n Wholesome Whole Wheat Recipe Fried Chicken.

FROZEN ENTRÉE: POT PIE

PRODUCT: Banquet Chicken Pie

INGREDIENTS: Filling: chicken broth, chicken roll, chicken meat, soy protein concentrate, salt, water, sodium phosphate, cellulose gum, water, chicken skin, starch, potatoes, flour, carrots, peas, salt, flavorings, vegetable oil, monosodium glutamate, beta carotene, paprika, oleoresin of turmeric, dextrose, disodium inosinate, disodium guanylate. Crust: enriched flour (wheat flour, niacin, ferrous sulfate, thiamine hydrochloride, riboflavin), shortening, water, dextrose, salt, sodium bicarbonate, sodium aluminum phosphate, nonfat dry milk, artificial color, FD&C Yellow No. 5.

NUTRITION PER SERVING: 8 ounce serving; 520 calories; 16 g protein; 45 g carbohydrate; 30 g* fat; 1,027 mg* sodium.

PRODUCTS TO REPLACE: All major brands, including: Morton; Stouffer's.

REPLACEMENT: Swanson Chicken Pot Pie

INGREDIENTS: Chicken broth, enriched wheat flour, cooked chicken meat, shortening, water, carrots, dehydrated potatoes, chicken, chicken skins, wheat flour, chicken fat, modified food starch, margarine, peas, salt, dextrose, whey powder, sweet peppers, monosodium glutamate, dehydrated onions, lactic acid, spice, celery seeds.

NUTRITION PER SERVING: 8 ounce serving; 420 calories; 13 g protein; 39 g carbohydrate; 24 g* fat; 850 mg* sodium.

ENTRÉE: SPAGHETTI

Most packaged frozen dinners contain refined sweeteners, preservatives, and artificial ingredients. Even so, some choices are much better than others.

PRODUCT: Weight Watchers Spaghetti with Meat Sauce

INGREDIENTS: Cooked enriched spaghetti, tomato puree, cooked beef, tomatoes, mushrooms, burgundy wine flavor, modified food starch, sugar, salt, dehydrated onions, corn oil, Romano cheese, olive oil, spice, monosodium glutamate, granulated garlic, calcium chloride, citric acid.

NUTRITION PER SERVING: 10.5 ounce serving; 280 calories; 20 g protein; 32 g carbohydrate, 7 g fat, 610 mg* sodium.

PRODUCTS TO REPLACE: Most major brands, including: Lean Cuisine; Stouffer's.

REPLACEMENT: Healthy Choice Spaghetti with Meat Sauce

INGREDIENTS: Meat sauce: tomatoes, beef, mushrooms, sugar, dehydrated onions, soybean oil, Parmesan cheese, flavorings, salt, spices, lemon juice. Spaghetti: cooked spaghetti noodles, soybean oil.

NUTRITION PER SERVING: 10 ounce serving; 280 calories; 14 g protein; 47 g carbohydrate; 4 g fat; 260 mg sodium.

OTHER REPLACEMENTS: Swanson Spaghetti in Tomato Sauce with Breaded Veal; Ultra Slim Fast Spaghetti with Beef and Mushroom Sauce.

FROZEN ENTRÉE: LASAGNA

PRODUCT: Stouffer's Lean Cuisine Lasagna

INGREDIENTS: Tomatoes, beef, cooked macaroni product, low-moisture part-skim cheese, tomato puree, onions, dry curd cottage cheese, tomatoes with puree, water, mushrooms, celery, modified cornstarch, tomato paste, Parmesan cheese, salt, sugar, enriched flour, Romano cheese, spices, xanthan gum, mushroom base (sauteed mushrooms, salt, monosodium glutamate, sugar, butter), hydrolyzed vegetable protein, sugar cane syrup, cooked chicken, monosodium glutamate, dehydrated garlic, chicken fat, corn oil, dehydrated onions, caramel coloring, natural flavorings, dried beef stock, chicken broth, turmeric.

NUTRITION PER SERVING: 10.25 ounce serving size; 270 calories; 25 g protein; 24 g carbohydrate; 8 g fat; 970 mg* sodium.

PRODUCTS TO REPLACE: Most major brands, including: Budget Gourmet Light, Le Menu Light; Stouffer's; Weight Watchers.

REPLACEMENT: Celentano Lasagna

INGREDIENTS: Tomatoes, ricotta, unbleached enriched durum wheat flour, mozzarella, eggs, water, Romano cheese, peanut oil, garlic, onion, oregano, basil, parsley, salt, pepper.

NUTRITION PER SERVING: 7 ounce serving; 288 calories; 14 g protein; 31 g carbohydrate; 12 g* fat; 600 mg* sodium.

OTHER REPLACEMENTS: Celentano Broccoli Stuffed Shells; Celentano Cheese Ravioli; Healthy Choice.

BE ON THE LOOKOUT FOR: Legume lasagna and frozen food entrées. This brand has no refined sweeteners, artificial ingredients, or preservatives; it is low in fat and calories, and relatively low in sodium. They offer other Italian meals, manicotti and stuffed shells, as well as Mexican entrées.

PIZZA

PRODUCT: Stouffer's French Bread Cheese Pizza

INGREDIENTS: French bread (bleached enriched flour [wheat flour, niacin, iron, thiamine mononitrate, riboflavin], water, corn syrup, salt, yeast, vegetable shortening [partially hydrogenated soybean, cottonseed and/or palm oil], corn sugar, dough conditioners [vegetable mono- and diglycerides, vegetable calcium stearoyl-2-lactylate, monocalcium phosphate, calcium sulfate, ammonium sulfate, potassium bromate], calcium propionate, cornstarch, soy flour, acetic acid, lactic acid), tomatoes, low-moisture part-skim mozzarella cheese, tomato puree, brick cheese, margarine (partially hydrogenated soybean oil, skim milk, salt, vegetable lecithin, vegetable mono- and diglycerides, sodium benzoate and citric acid, artificial flavor, beta carotene, vitamin A palmitate), tomato paste, Parmesan cheese, corn oil, sugar, modified cornstarch, Romano cheese, salt, dehydrated onions, spices, beef, erythorbic acid, dehydrated garlic, natural flavors, monosodium glutamate, caramel coloring, dried beef stock.

NUTRITION PER SERVING: 1 slice serving; 330 calories; 10 g protein; 43 g carbohydrate; 13 g* fat; 850 mg* sodium.

PRODUCTS TO REPLACE: All major brands.

REPLACEMENT: Celentano Thick Crust Pizza

INGREDIENTS: Topping: Tomatoes, mozzarella cheese, peanut oil, salt, oregano, onion, garlic, parsley, basil, pepper. Crust: Unbleached enriched flour, water, vegetable shortening, yeast.

NUTRITION PER SERVING: ⅓ pie serving; 238 calories; 13 g protein; 31 g carbohydrate; 7 g fat; 252 mg sodium.

OTHER REPLACEMENTS: Celentano Nine Slice Pizza; Tree Tavern.

BE ON THE LOOKOUT FOR: Graindance pizzas.

BEVERAGES: JUICE BLENDS; JUICE SPRITZERS; PUNCH-TYPE DRINKS; CARBONATED BEVERAGES/ SODAS; MILK PRODUCTS; COCOA; COFFEE/TEA/ ICED TEA

We don't do a comparison for straight juices, like orange juice or apple juice, because, fortunately, many of these products are 100% juice. It's in some of the other exploding growth categories—like juice blends/drinks and spritzers—where things get murkier. Our comparisons follow.

JUICE BLENDS

PRODUCT: Ocean Spray Cranapple Cranberry Apple Drink

INGREDIENTS: Filtered water, high fructose corn syrup, cranberry juice (cranberry juice, cranberry juice concentrate), apple juice from concentrate, natural flavors, fumaric acid, ascorbic acid.

NUTRITION PER SERVING: 6 fluid ounce serving; 130 calories; 0 g protein, 3 g carbohydrate, 0 g fat, 10 mg sodium.

PRODUCTS TO REPLACE: Any major brands containing refined sweeteners or additives, including: Kern's Nectars—Apple Strawberry, Banana Pineapple, Orange Banana, Strawberry Banana; Ocean Spray drinks—Crangrape, Cranraspberry, Cranstrawberry; Sunny Delight Florida Citrus Punch; Tropicana Twister Fruit Beverages—Orange Cranberry, Orange Passionfruit, Orange Peach, Orange Raspberry.

REPLACEMENT: Smucker's Apple Cranberry

INGREDIENTS: Water, concentrated white grape, apple, peach, red raspberry, and red currant juices, natural flavors.

NUTRITION PER SERVING: 8 ounce serving; 120 calories; 0 g protein; 32 g carbohydrate; 0 g fat; 10 mg sodium.

OTHER REPLACEMENTS: Any brands without sugar and additives, including: Chiquita Juice Blends (in refrigerator section)—Caribbean Splash, Island Orchard, Orange Banana, Tropical Squeeze; Dole Pure and Light Juice Blends (in refrigerator section)—Country Raspberry, Mandarin Tangerine, Mountain Cherry, Orchard Peach, Pineapple Orange Guava, Pineapple Orange Banana; all R. W. Knudsen Juice blends; Tree Top Juice Blends—Apple Cranberry, Apple Pear, Apple Grape.)

JUICE SPRITZERS

PRODUCT: Tropicana Juice Sparkler

INGREDIENTS: Grape juice concentrate; sparkling water, berry flavors, high fructose corn syrup, ascorbic acid.

NUTRITION PER SERVING: 8 fluid ounce serving; 75 calories; 0 g protein; 16 g carbohydrate; 0 g fat; 16 mg sodium.

PRODUCTS TO REPLACE: Most major brands, including: Tropicana Juice Sparklers; Wallaroo Natural Sparklers.

REPLACEMENT: Sundance Natural Cranberry Sparkler

INGREDIENTS: White grape and cranberry juice from concentrate, sparkling water, natural flavors.

NUTRITION PER SERVING: 10 fluid ounce serving; 133 calories; less than 1 g protein; 32 g carbohydrate; 0 g fat; 29 mg sodium.

OTHER REPLACEMENTS: R. W. Knudsen Fruit Juice Spritzers—Black Cherry, Orange Passionfruit, Peach, Tangerine; Sundance Natural Sparklers—all flavors.

PUNCH-TYPE DRINKS

PRODUCT: Hi-C Cherry

INGREDIENTS: Water, high fructose corn syrup, grape and cherry juices from concentrate, sugar, fumaric acid, citric acid, ascorbic acid, artificial colors, natural flavor.

NUTRITION PER SERVING: 6 fluid ounce serving; 100 calories; 0 g protein; 25 g carbohydrates; 0 g fat; 25 mg sodium.

PRODUCTS TO REPLACE: Most major brands, including: CapriSun 100% Naturals—Orange, Red Berry, Maui Punch; Hawaiian Punch Fruit Juicy Red Punch;

Hi-C—all flavors; Minute Maid 100% Natural Fruit Punch; Sunny Delight Florida Citrus Punch.

REPLACEMENT: Libby's Juicy Juice Cherry

INGREDIENTS: Apple, grape, and cherry juices from concentrate, natural flavors, vitamin C.

NUTRITION PER SERVING: 6 fluid ounce serving; 90 calories; 1 g protein; 23 g carbohydrate; 0 g fat; 10 mg sodium.

OTHER REPLACEMENTS: Libby's Juicy Juice—Berry, Punch, Tropical grape.

CARBONATED BEVERAGES (SODAS): LEMON LIME

PRODUCT: Diet 7-Up

INGREDIENTS: Carbonated water, citric acid, aspartame (NutraSweet brand), sodium benzoate, sodium citrate, lemon and lime flavors.

NUTRITION PER SERVING: 6 ounce fluid serving; 2 calories; 0 g protein; 0 g carbohydrates; 0 g fat; 35 mg sodium.

PRODUCTS TO REPLACE: All major brands, including: Diet Lemon Lime Slice; Diet Mountain Dew; Diet Sprite; Diet Squirt; Hansen's Natural Lemon Lime Soda; Lemon Lime Slice; Mountain Dew; 7-Up; Shasta Diet Lemon Lime; Sprite; Squirt.

REPLACEMENT: Canada Dry Sparkling Water Lemon Lime

INGREDIENTS: Carbonated water, natural flavors.

NUTRITION PER SERVING: 6 ounce serving; 0 calories; 0 g protein; 0 g carbohydrate; 0 g fat; 0 g sodium.

OTHER REPLACEMENTS: Any brand without refined or artificial sweeteners or additives, including: Perrier with Natural Lemon; Perrier with Natural Lime.

CARBONATED BEVERAGES (SODAS): ORANGE

PRODUCT: Diet Sunkist Orange Soda

> **INGREDIENTS:** Carbonated water, citric acid, sodium citrate, aspartame (NutraSweet brand), modified food starch and/or gum acacia, sodium benzoate, ascorbic acid, malic acid, natural flavors, caffeine, FD&C Yellow No. 6, glycerol ester of wood rosin.

> **NUTRITION PER SERVING:** 6 ounce serving; 2 calories; 0 g protein; 0 g carbohydrate; 0 g fat; 65 mg sodium.

> **PRODUCTS TO REPLACE:** Most major brands, including: Diet Minute Maid Orange Soda; Diet Slice Mandarin Orange; Hansen's Mandarin Orange Natural Soda; Minute Maid Orange Soda; Shasta Orange Soda; Slice Mandarin Orange; Sunkist Orange Soda.

REPLACEMENT: Canada Dry Natural Mandarin Orange Seltzer

> **INGREDIENTS:** Carbonated water, natural flavors.

> **NUTRITION PER SERVING:** 6 ounce serving; 0 calories; 0 g protein; 0 g carbohydrate; 0 g fat; 0 g sodium.

> **OTHER REPLACEMENTS:** Perrier with Natural Orange; R. W. Knudsen Orange Soda.

CARBONATED BEVERAGES (SODA): COLAS

Even though most sodas contain acids, refined sweeteners or artificial sweeteners, and/or caffeine, you can make choices that will leave some of these additives behind.

PRODUCT: Dr. Pepper

INGREDIENTS: Carbonated water, sugar and/or corn sweetener, caramel color, artificial and natural flavoring, phosphoric acid, sodium benzoate, caffeine, monosodium phosphate, lactic acid, polyethylene glycol.

NUTRITION PER SERVING: 12 ounce serving; 159 calories; 0 g protein; 41 g carbohydrate; 0 g fat; 36 mg sodium.

PRODUCTS TO REPLACE: Most major caffeinated brands.

REPLACEMENT: Caffeine-free Coca-Cola

INGREDIENTS: Carbonated water, high fructose corn syrup and/or sucrose, caramel color, phosphoric acid, natural flavors.

NUTRITION PER SERVING: 12 ounce serving; 144 calories; 0 g protein; 38 g carbohydrate; 1 g fat; 22 mg sodium.

MILK PRODUCTS

PRODUCT: Carnation Evaporated Milk

INGREDIENTS: Milk, disodium phosphate, carrageenan, vitamin D_3.

NUTRITION PER SERVING: ½ cup serving; 170 calories; 8 g protein; 12 g carbohydrate; 10 g fat; 133 mg sodium.

REPLACEMENT: Carnation Evaporated Skimmed Milk

INGREDIENTS: Skimmed milk, vitamin A palmitate, vitamin D_3.

NUTRITION PER SERVING: ½ cup serving; 100 calories; 9 g protein; 14 g carbohydrate; less than 1 g fat; 15 mg sodium.

OTHER REPLACEMENTS: Carnation Instant Nonfat Dry Milk.

COCOA

All major brands—regular or diet—of cocoa mixes have sugar or artificial sweeteners and additives. *Recommendation:* Use sparingly.

> *BE ON THE LOOKOUT FOR:* Vitasoy Rich Cocoa. This brand, being introduced to supermarkets, has no refined sugars or additives.

COFFEE/TEA/ICED TEA

Picking a decaffeinated coffee or tea—regardless of brand—over a caffeinated brand is always a good choice. When it comes to iced tea, however, there can be differences among products.

PRODUCT: Sugarfree Nestea Decaf

INGREDIENTS: Maltodextrin, decaffeinated instant tea, malic acid, aspartame (NutraSweet brand), gum arabic, natural lemon flavors.

NUTRITION PER SERVING: 2 tsp. serving; 0 calories; 0 g protein; 1 g carbohydrate; 0 g fat; 0 mg sodium.

PRODUCTS TO REPLACE: All brands with artificial sweeteners and additives, including: Lipton Natural Decaffeinated Sugarfree Iced Tea.

REPLACEMENT: Lipton Instant Naturally Decaffeinated Tea

INGREDIENTS: Decaffeinated instant tea.

NUTRITION PER SERVING: 2 tsp. serving size; 0 calories; 0 g protein; 0 g carbohydrate; 0 g fat; 0 mg sodium.

BREAD/ENGLISH MUFFINS/ CROUTONS/MEAT-POULTRY COATING/STUFFING

. . . .

BREAD: WHITE OR EGG

Local bakeries may provide good sugar-free, additive-free whole grain bread choices. Most major brands of bread are enriched and do contain additives. However, as the following comparisons show, some products stand out over others when it comes to their ingredients.

PRODUCT: Wonder Bread

INGREDIENTS: Enriched flour (barley malt, iron [ferrous sulfate], niacin, thiamine mononitrate, riboflavin), water, corn syrup, yeast, vegetable oil (may contain soybean and/or corn and/or cottonseed and/or canola oil), salt, wheat gluten, soy flour, calcium sulfate, dough conditioners (contains one or more of the following: sodium stearoyl lactylate, mono- and diglycerides, mono- or dicalcium phosphate), potassium bromate.

NUTRITION PER SERVING: 1 slice serving; 60 calories; 2 g protein; 10 g carbohydrate; 1 g fat; 120 mg sodium.

PRODUCTS TO REPLACE: Most major brands, including: Home Pride Butter Top White; Weber's.

REPLACEMENT: Arnold Brick Oven White Bread

INGREDIENTS: Unbleached enriched wheat flour (flour, malted barley flour, niacin, reduced iron, thiamine mononitrate, riboflavin), water, corn syrup, partially hydrogenated soybean oil, salt, whey, yeast, nonfat milk, soy flour, mono- and diglycerides, honey, butter.

NUTRITION PER SERVING: 2 slice serving; 130 calories; 4 g protein; 22 g carbohydrate; 2 g fat; 205 mg sodium.

OTHER REPLACEMENTS: Pepperidge Farm White Thin Sliced Bread.

BE ON THE LOOKOUT FOR: Good Stuff Egg Sesame Bread.

BREAD: WHEAT/WHOLE GRAIN/BRAN

PRODUCT: Roman Meal Bread

INGREDIENTS: Bleached wheat flour, water, corn syrup, select wheat bran, whole wheat, soybean oil, whole rye, honey, molasses, yeast, salt, soy flour, wheat gluten, whey solids, calcium sulfate, dough conditioners (sodium stearoyl, lactylate, malted barley flour, potassium bromate), defatted flaxseed meal, ammonium sulfate, calcium propionate, ferrous sulfate, niacin, thiamine mononitrate, riboflavin.

NUTRITION PER SERVING: 1 slice serving; 70 calories; 3 g protein; 13 g carbohydrate; 1 g fat; 140 mg sodium.

PRODUCTS TO REPLACE: Most major brands, including: Homepride Butter Top Seven Grain; Homepride Buttertop Wheat; Millbrook Autumn Grain; Millbrook Cracked Wheat; Oroweat Breads—Health Nut; Honey Wheat Berry; Oatnut; Whole Wheat; Pepperidge Farm Honey Wheat Berry Bread; Weber Light Wheat; Wonder Light Wheat.

REPLACEMENT: Arnold Brick Oven Whole Wheat Bread

INGREDIENTS: Whole wheat flour, water, corn syrup, partially hydrogenated soybean oil, molasses, salt, yeast, wheat gluten, whey, soy flour, ethoxylated mono- and diglycerides.

NUTRITION PER SERVING: 2 slice serving; 120 calories; 4 g protein; 19 g carbohydrate; 3 g fat; 190 mg sodium.

OTHER REPLACEMENTS: Arnold Honey Wheat Berry; Arnold Original Bran'nola; Pritikin Stone Ground Whole Wheat.

BE ON THE LOOKOUT FOR: Food for Life, Good Stuff, and Grainsworth breads.

ENGLISH MUFFINS

PRODUCT: Thomas' English Muffins

INGREDIENTS: Enriched wheat flour (unbleached wheat flour, malted barley, niacin, reduced iron, thiamine mononitrate, riboflavin), water, farina, corn syrup, yeast, salt, partially hydrogenated soybean oil, mono- and diglycerides, whey solids, vinegar, calcium propionate.

NUTRITION PER SERVING: 1 muffin serving; 130 calories; 4 g protein; 25 g carbohydrate; 1 g fat; 200 mg sodium.

PRODUCTS TO REPLACE: Most major brands, including: Oatmeal Goodness English Muffins; Pepperidge Farm English Muffins; Roman Meal English Muffins; Sun Maid Raisin Muffins; Weber's Oat Bran Muffins.

REPLACEMENT: Pritikin English Muffins

> INGREDIENTS: Water, whole wheat, wheat grits, wheat gluten, yeast, raisin juice concentrate, yellow corn flour, cultured whey, salt, ascorbic acid.

> NUTRITION PER SERVING: 1 muffin serving; 135 calories; 9 g protein; 25 g carbohydrate; 2 g fat; 140 mg sodium.

> *BE ON THE LOOKOUT FOR:* Good Stuff Whole Grain English Muffins and Good Stuff Whole Grain Raisin Nut Muffins.

CROUTONS

Most major brands of croutons are enriched and have lots of additives and preservatives. However, as follows, there is a choice you can make that will leave lots of those additives out of your salads.

PRODUCT: Mrs. Cubbison's Cool Herb Restaurant-Style Croutons

> INGREDIENTS: Enriched flour, water, partially hydrogenated soybean oil, cultured buttermilk, salt, corn syrup, soy flour, yeast, whey, tomato powder, dehydrated onions and garlic, calcium sulfate, natural and artificial flavors, Cheddar cheese (cultured milk, salt, calcium chloride, enzymes, disodium phosphate, monosodium glutamate, sugar, parsley, dextrose, spices, calcium propionate, malic, citric, and lactic acids, sodium casseinate, sodium diacetate, disodium inosinate, disodium guanylate, artificial color, FD&C Yellow No. 5.

> NUTRITION PER SERVING: ½ cup serving; 130 calories; 3 g protein; 16 g carbohydrate; 5 g fat; 430 mg* sodium.

PRODUCTS TO REPLACE: All major brands.

REPLACEMENT: Pepperidge Farm Cheddar and Romano Cheese Croutons

INGREDIENTS: Unbleached enriched wheat flour, vegetable oil, dehydrated Cheddar cheese, water, corn syrup, salt, dehydrated Romano cheese, yeast, vinegar, natural flavor, citric acid.

NUTRITION PER SERVING: ½ cup serving; 120 calories; 4 g protein; 18 g carbohydrate; 4 g fat; 380 mg sodium.

MEAT/POULTRY/CHOPS COATING MIX

PRODUCT: Shake 'n Bake Original Recipe Chicken

INGREDIENTS: Bleached bromated wheat flour, dextrin, partially hydrogenated soybean and cottonseed oils, salt, paprika, malted barley, spices (mustard flour, celery seed, chili pepper, black pepper, thyme, basil, red pepper, cloves, oregano, rosemary), sugar, yeast, beet powder, garlic powder, onion powder, hickory smoke flavor, TBHQ, calcium propionate.

NUTRITION PER SERVING: 2 chicken pieces coated serving; 80 calories; 2 g protein; 14 g carbohydrate; 2 g fat; 450 mg* sodium.

PRODUCTS TO REPLACE: All major brands.

REPLACEMENT: Kellogg's Corn Flake Crumbs for Chicken, Chops, Meat Loaf, and Desserts

INGREDIENTS: Corn, sugar, salt, malt flavoring, corn syrup.

NUTRITION PER SERVING: 1 ounce serving; 100 calories; 2 g protein; 24 g carbohydrate; 0 g fat; 290 mg sodium.

BE ON THE LOOKOUT FOR: El Molino Unprocessed Miller's Bran Flakes for Meat and Poultry Coating.

STUFFING

All major brands of stuffing mix are enriched and many have a laundry list of additives. You can make a choice, though, that will put many fewer additives and preservatives on your table.

PRODUCT: Stove Top Stuffing Mix

INGREDIENTS: Enriched bromated wheat flour (niacin, iron, thiamine mononitrate, riboflavin), corn syrup, salt, onion, partially hydrogenated soybean and/or cottonseed oils, yeast, celery, turkey broth, hydrolyzed vegetable protein, soy flour, whey, parsley flakes, calcium propionate, sodium sulfite, BHA, TBHQ, citric acid, propyl gallate, caramel color, sugar, onion powder, disodium inosinate, disodium guanylate, turmeric.

NUTRITION PER SERVING: ½ cup (dry mix) serving; 110 calories; 4 g protein; 21 g carbohydrate; 1 g fat; 560 mg* sodium.

PRODUCTS TO REPLACE: All major brands.

REPLACEMENT: Pepperidge Farm Seasoned Stuffing Mix

INGREDIENTS: Unbleached enriched wheat flour, whole wheat flour, water, salt, corn syrup, yeast, partially hydrogenated vegetable shortening, molasses, spices, onion powder, calcium propionate, celery seed, mono- and diglycerides, citric acid.

NUTRITION PER SERVING: ½ cup serving; 134 calories; 4 g protein; 22 g carbohydrate; 2 g fat; 400 mg sodium.

BE ON THE LOOKOUT FOR: Shelton's Blue Corn and Cornbread Dressings.

CEREAL (COLD/HOT)/ GRANOLA BARS

CEREAL—COLD: FLAKE CEREALS

PRODUCT: General Mills' Wheaties

> **INGREDIENTS:** Whole wheat, sugar, salt, malt extract, corn syrup, calcium carbonate, calcium chloride, trisodium phosphate, sodium ascorbate, niacinamide, iron, palmitate, pyridoxine hydrochloride, riboflavin, thiamine mononitrate, folic acid, vitamin D, BHT.

> **NUTRITION PER SERVING:** 1 ounce serving; 100 calories; 3 g protein; 23 g carbohydrate; 1 g fat; 200 mg sodium.

> **PRODUCTS TO REPLACE:** Any major brand containing refined sweetener and/or additives and preservatives, including: General Mills' Wheat and Bran Clusters; Kellogg's cereals—Bran Flakes; Common Sense; Corn Flakes; Heartwise; Just Right; Product 19; Post Oat Flakes; Team; Total.

REPLACEMENT: Kellogg's Nutri-Grain Wheat Flakes

> **INGREDIENTS:** Whole wheat kernels, malt flavoring, salt.

> **NUTRITION PER SERVING:** 1 ounce serving; 90 calories; 3 g protein; 23 g carbohydrate; 0 g fat; 170 mg sodium.

OTHER REPLACEMENTS: Health Valley cereals—Oat Bran O's; Organic Fiber Seven Flakes; Organic Oat Bran Flakes; Uncle Sam Toasted Whole Grain Wheat Flakes.

BE ON THE LOOKOUT FOR: Grainfield's Corn Flakes; Manna Multigrain Oatbran Flakes.

CEREAL—COLD: RAISIN BRANS

PRODUCT: General Mills' Total Raisin Bran

INGREDIENTS: Wheat bran and other parts of wheat, raisins, sugar, tricalcium and dicalcium phosphate, brown sugar, syrup, salt, corn syrup, malt syrup, honey, zinc, iron, tocopheryl acetate, niacinamide, trisodium calcium pantothenate, palmitate, pyridox hydrochloride, riboflavin, thiamine mononitrate, folic acid, vitamin B_{12}, vitamin D, BHT.

NUTRITION PER SERVING: 1.5 ounce serving; 140 calories; 3 g protein; 33 g carbohydrate; 1 g fat; 190 mg sodium.

PRODUCTS TO REPLACE: Most major brands, including: General Mills' Oatmeal Raisin Crisp; General Mills' Raisin Nut Bran; Kellogg's Raisin Bran; Post Raisin Bran.

REPLACEMENT: Kellogg's Nutri-Grain Raisin Bran

INGREDIENTS: Whole wheat, raisins, wheat bran, malt flavoring, glycerin, salt.

NUTRITION PER SERVING: 1.4 ounce serving; 140 calories; 3 g protein; 31 g carbohydrate; 2 g fat; 220 mg sodium.

OTHER REPLACEMENTS: Kellogg's Nutri-Grain Almond Raisin.

BE ON THE LOOKOUT FOR: Grainfield's Whole Grain Raisin Bran; Manna Raisin and Oat Bran.

CEREAL—COLD: ASSORTED VARIETIES

PRODUCT: Apple Cinnamon Cheerios

INGREDIENTS: Whole oat flour, sugar, dried apple pieces, corn syrup, partially hydrogenated soybean oil, wheat starch, salt, cinnamon, calcium carbonate, trisodium phosphate, sodium sulfite, sulfur dioxide, BHT.

NUTRITION PER SERVING: 1 ounce serving; 110 calories; 2 g protein; 22 g carbohydrate; 2 g fat; 180 mg sodium.

PRODUCTS TO REPLACE: Most major brands, including: Cheerios; Chex cereals; Honey Nut Cheerios; Kellogg's Nut and Honey Crunch O's; Kix; Life.

REPLACEMENT: Nabisco Shredded Wheat

INGREDIENTS: Whole wheat.

NUTRITION PER SERVING: ⅔ cup serving; 90 calories; 3 g protein; 23 g carbohydrate; 0 g fat; 0 mg sodium.

OTHER REPLACEMENTS: Any unenriched brand with no refined sweeteners, additives, or preservatives, including: Health Valley cereals: Post Grape Nuts; Malt-O-Meal Puffed Rice; Nabisco Shredded Wheat with Oat Bran; Outrageous Fruit and Grains.

CEREAL—HOT

PRODUCT: Instant Quaker Oatmeal Peaches and Cream

INGREDIENTS: Rolled oats, sugar, creaming agent (maltodextrin, partially hydrogenated soybean oil, skim milk solids), flavored fruit pieces (dehydrated apples, sulfur dioxide, sodium sulfite, sodium bisulfite), dehydrated peaches, artificial flavor, citric acid, annatto, salt, calcium carbonate, guar gum, artificial flavors, vitamin A palmitate, reduced iron, niacinamide, pyroxine hydrochloride, thiamine mononitrate, riboflavin, folic acid.

NUTRITION PER SERVING: 1.25 ounce serving; 130 calories; 3 g protein; 26 g carbohydrate; 2 g fat; 180 mg sodium.

PRODUCTS TO REPLACE: Most major brands, including: General Mills' Oatmeal Swirlers varieties; Instant Cream of Wheat varieties; Instant Quaker Oatmeal varieties; Instant Total Oatmeal varieties; Quick Cream of Wheat; Quick Malt-O-Meal.

REPLACEMENT: Quick Quaker Oats

INGREDIENTS: Rolled oats.

NUTRITION PER SERVING: 1 ounce serving; 100 calories; 5 g protein; 18 g carbohydrate; 2 g fat; 0 mg sodium.

OTHER REPLACEMENTS: Any unenriched brands with no refined sweeteners, additives or preservatives, including: Quaker Oat Bran Hot Cereal; Roman Meal Oats, Wheat, Rye Bran Flax; Wheatena.

GRANOLA BARS

PRODUCT: Quaker Chewy Granola Bars

INGREDIENTS: Granola (rolled oats, rolled whole wheat, brown sugar, partially hydrogenated vegetable oil [soybean and/or cottonseed oil], nonfat dry milk, dried unsweetened coconut, honey), crisp rice (rice, sugar, salt, malt), semisweet chocolate chips (sugar, chocolate liqueur, cocoa butter, lecithin, vanilla flavor), invert sugar, peanut butter (peanuts, sucrose, hydrogenated vegetable oil [cottonseed and/or rapeseed oil], salt), peanut-butter-flavored chips (partially defatted peanut meal, sugar, partially hydrogenated vegetable oil [soybean and cottonseed], lecithin, artificial flavor), peanuts, corn syrup solids, glycerin, honey, sorbitol, salt, citric acid.

NUTRITION PER SERVING: 1 bar serving; 130 calories; 3 g protein; 17 g carbohydrate; 6 g fat; 110 mg sodium.

PRODUCTS TO REPLACE: All major brands, including: Carnation Breakfast Bar varieties; Kellogg's Smart Start Cereal Bars varieties; Kudos Bars varieties; Quaker Chewy Granola Bars varieties; Quaker Granola Dips varieties.

REPLACEMENT: Nature's Choice Fresh and Chewy Granola Bars, Peanut Butter

INGREDIENTS: Granola (rolled oats, honey, canola oil), honey, peanuts, brown rice, malted cereals (corn, barley), peanut butter, canola oil, natural flavor, lecithin.

NUTRITION PER SERVING: 1 bar serving; 90 calories; 2 g protein; 14 g carbohydrate; 4 g fat; 25 mg sodium.

OTHER REPLACEMENTS: Health Valley Cholesterol Free—Fat Free Apple Fruit Bars, Apricot Fruit Bars, Date Fruit Bars; Nature's Choice Fresh and Chewy Granola Bars—all varieties.

CRACKERS

WHEAT VARIETIES

PRODUCT: Nabisco Wheat Thins

INGREDIENTS: Wheat flour, enriched wheat flour (niacin, reduced iron, thiamine mononitrate, riboflavin), vegetable shortening (partially hydrogenated soybean oil), sugar, salt, high fructose corn syrup, malted barley flour, annatto extract, turmeric, paprika oleoresins.

NUTRITION PER SERVING: ½ ounce serving; 70 calories; 1 g protein; 9 g carbohydrate; 3 g fat; 120 mg sodium.

PRODUCTS TO REPLACE: Most major brands, including: Keebler Wheatables Whole Wheat Crackers; Nabisco Triscuits Whole Wheat Wafers; Sunshine American Heritage Wheat Bran Crackers; Sunshine Hi Ho Deluxe Whole Wheat Crackers.

REPLACEMENT: Health Valley Stoned Ground Wheat Crackers

INGREDIENTS: Wheat flour, safflower oil, cracked wheat, malt, sea salt, yeast.

NUTRITION PER SERVING: ½ ounce serving; 55 calories; 1 g protein; 9 g carbohydrate; 2 g fat; 30 mg sodium.

GRAIN CRACKERS

PRODUCT: Pepperidge Farm Distinctive Sesame Crackers

INGREDIENTS: Unbleached wheat flour, whole wheat flour, nonfat milk, partially hydrogenated vegetable shortening (canola, cottonseed and/or soybean oils), sesame seeds, defatted wheat germ, yeast, salt, baking soda, barley malt, brown sugar, garlic powder, dextrin.

NUTRITION PER SERVING: 4 cracker serving; 80 calories; 2 g protein; 12 g carbohydrate; 4 g fat; 140 mg sodium.

PRODUCTS TO REPLACE: Most major brands, including: Keebler Toasteds Sesame Crackers; Nabisco Ritz Crackers; Sunshine American Heritage Sesame Crackers.

REPLACEMENT: Ralston Natural Ry Krisp

INGREDIENTS: Whole rye, corn, bran, salt, caraway.

NUTRITION PER SERVING: ½ ounce serving; 40 calories; 1 g protein; 11 g carbohydrate; 0 g fat; 75 mg sodium.

OTHER REPLACEMENTS: Finn Crisp; Ideal Fiber Thins; Wasa—Light Rye, Sesame Rye, Sesame Wheat.

COOKIES
. . . .

More and more smaller company's brands of sugar-free or fruit-juice-sweetened cookies with no additives or artificial ingredients are appearing in supermarkets (see the BE ON THE LOOKOUT FOR listings throughout this section). Most major brands use enriched flour, refined sweeteners, preservatives, and artificial ingredients. As evidenced in the following comparisons, though, you can buy popular brands that use no artificial ingredients or preservatives.

CHOCOLATE OR CHIP COOKIES

PRODUCT: Nabisco Chips Ahoy! Selections Chocolate Chip Cookies

> **INGREDIENTS:** Enriched wheat flour (niacin, reduced iron, thiamine, mononitrate, riboflavin), vegetable shortening (partially hydrogenated soybean or cottonseed oil), sugar, bittersweet chocolate drops (sugar, chocolate, partially processed with alkali, cocoa butter, butteroil, soy lecithin, emulsifier, salt, artificial vanillin), walnuts, butter, cocoa (with alkali), eggs, skim milk, cocoa, leavening (baking soda, calcium phosphate), salt, corn syrup, natural and artificial flavor, chocolate and soy lecithin.

> **NUTRITION PER SERVING:** 1 cookie serving; 95 calories; 1 g protein; 9 g carbohydrate; 6 g fat; 70 mg sodium.

> **PRODUCTS TO REPLACE:** Most major brands, including: Chips Ahoy! Chocolate Chunk Pecan Oatmeal Chocolate Chunk; Famous Amos Chocolate Chip Cookies; Keebler Rainbow Chips Deluxe; Keebler Soft Batch Cookies; Mother's Chocolate Chip Cookies; Nabisco Oreo Chocolate Sandwich Cookies.

REPLACEMENT: Pepperidge Farm Chocolate-Laced Pirouettes

> **INGREDIENTS:** Unbleached wheat flour, sugar, partially hydrogenated vegetable shortening, sweet chocolate, egg whites, lecithin, nonfat milk, salt, vanilla extract.

> **NUTRITION PER SERVING:** 3 cookie serving; 110 calories; 0 g protein; 13 g carbohydrate; 7 g fat; 45 mg sodium.

OTHER REPLACEMENTS: Pepperidge Farm Milano Distinctive Cookies.

BE ON THE LOOKOUT FOR: Frookie Chocolate Chip Cookies; Nature's Warehouse—Carob Fudge, Chocolate Chocolate Chip Cookies, Oat Bran Chocolate Chip, Peanut Butter Chocolate Chip.

GRAIN OR FRUIT COOKIES

PRODUCT: Nabisco Fig Newtons Fruit Chewy Cookies

INGREDIENTS: Figs (sulfur dioxide), sugar, enriched wheat flour (niacin, reduced iron, thiamine mononitrate, riboflavin), corn syrup, vegetable shortening (partially hydrogenated soybean oil), high fructose corn syrup, salt, whey, yellow corn flour, baking soda, artificial flavor.

NUTRITION PER SERVING: 1 cookie serving; 60 calories; 1 g protein; 11 g carbohydrate; 1 g fat; 60 mg sodium.

PRODUCTS TO REPLACE: Most major brands, including: Mother's Bakery Wagon—Apple Filled Oatmeal, Date Filled Oatmeal, Raspberry Filled Oatmeal; Mother's Fig Bars; Nabisco—Apple Newtons, Raspberry Newtons, Strawberry Newtons; Sunshine Golden Fruit Biscuit Cookies.

REPLACEMENT: Pepperidge Farm Large Old Fashioned Granola Cookies

INGREDIENTS: Unbleached wheat flour, partially hydrogenated vegetable shortening, brown sugar, sugar, oatmeal, whole eggs, almonds, coconut, raisins, butter, dates, honey, baking soda, vanilla extracts, salt.

NUTRITION PER SERVING: 1 cookie serving; 120 calories; 1 g protein: 15 g carbohydrate; 3 g fat; 85 mg sodium.

OTHER REPLACEMENTS: Health Valley—Almond Date, Fruit and Nut Oat Bran, Fruit Jumbo Raisin Nut, Fruit Jumbo Tropical Fruit.

BE ON THE LOOKOUT FOR: Frookie—Apple Cinnamon Oatbran, Oatmeal Raisin; Marin Brand—Fig bars, Peach Apricot Fig Bars, Raisin Oatbran; Nature's Warehouse—Fig Bars, Raspberry Fig Bars.

SNACKS: CHIPS/POPCORN/ RAISINS/NUTS/CANDY

CHIPS: TORTILLA OR CORN CHIPS

PRODUCT: Doritos Brand Jumpin' Jack Tortilla Chips

INGREDIENTS: Corn, vegetable oil (one or more of the following oils: corn, canola, sunflower, cottonseed, partially hydrogenated sunflower and/or partially hydrogenated soybean), sour cream (cultured cream, nonfat milk), whey, salt, Cheddar cheese (milk, cheese, culture, salt, calcium chloride, enzymes), maltodextrin, imitation parsley (cornstarch, gum arabic, gelatin, artificial colors, glycerol, extractives of turmeric), natural flavors, monosodium glutamate, onion powder, yeast extract, artificial flavor, citric acid, garlic powder, lactic acid, modified food starch, artificial color, spice, disodium inosinate, disodium guanylate.

NUTRITION PER SERVING: 1 ounce serving; 140 calories; 2 g protein; 18 g carbohydrate; 7 g fat; 220 mg sodium.

PRODUCTS TO REPLACE: Any major brand with artificial ingredients or preservatives, including: Doritos brand chips—Cool Ranch Flavor, Nacho Cheese Flavor, Salsa Rio Flavor; Laura Scudder's Restaurant Style Picante Flavor Tortilla Strips.

REPLACEMENT: Fritos Corn Chips

INGREDIENTS: Corn, vegetable oil (corn, peanut, soybean, sunflower, partially hydrogenated sunflower), salt.

NUTRITION PER SERVING: 1 ounce serving; 150 calories; 2 g protein; 16 g carbohydrate; 9 g fat; 220 mg sodium.

OTHER REPLACEMENTS: Doritos Toasted Corn Lightly Salted Tortilla Chips; Eagle Brand Tortilla Strips; Laura Scudder's Original or Restaurant Style Tortilla Chips.

CHIPS: CHEESE PUFFS

PRODUCT: Chee-tos Brand Puffs Cheese Flavored Snacks

INGREDIENTS: Enriched cornmeal (cornmeal, ferrous sulfate, niacin, thiamine mononitrate, riboflavin), vegetable oil (contains one or more of the following: partially hydrogenated canola oil, partially hydrogenated sunflower oil, partially hydrogenated peanut oil and/or partially hydrogenated cottonseed oil), whey, Cheddar cheese (milk, cheese culture, salt, enzymes, calcium chloride), salt, maltodextrin, sour cream, artificial flavor, monosodium glutamate, lactic acid, artificial colors, spice, citric acid.

NUTRITION PER SERVING: 1 ounce serving; 160 calories; 1 g protein; 16 g carbohydrate; 10 g* fat; 330 mg sodium.

PRODUCTS TO REPLACE: All major brands.

REPLACEMENT: Health Valley Cheddar Lites

INGREDIENTS: Cornmeal, safflower oil, sunflower oil, Cheddar cheese, sea salt.

NUTRITION PER SERVING: ¼ ounce serving; 40 calories; 1 g protein; 4 g carbohydrate; 2 g fat; 35 mg sodium.

BE ON THE LOOKOUT FOR: Bearitos Baked Cheddar Puffs; Skinny Haven Nacho Cheese Skinny Munchies.

POPCORN

PRODUCT: Keebler Pop Deluxe White Cheddar (Gourmet-Style Popcorn)

INGREDIENTS: Popcorn, vegetable oil (corn oil and partially hydrogenated soybean oil, TBHQ), dehydrated Cheddar, Parmesan and blue cheeses (milk, cheese cultures, salt, enzymes), whey, salt, maltodextrin, dehydrated sour cream, buttermilk, reduced lactose whey, nonfat dry milk, dehydrated butter, disodium phosphate, citric acid, artificial colors (contains FD&C Yellow No. 5 and No. 6), artificial flavor, lactic acid, natural flavor, monosodium glutamate, tricalcium phosphate.

NUTRITION PER SERVING: 1 ounce serving; 140 calories; 1 g protein; 13 g carbohydrate; 10 g* fat; 270 mg sodium.

PRODUCTS TO REPLACE: Any brand containing refined sweeteners, additives, or preservatives, including: Cape Cod Popcorn with White Cheddar Cheese; Keebler Pop Deluxe Honey Caramel Glazed Gourmet-Style Popcorn.

REPLACEMENT: Borden Wise Choice Premium White Cheddar Popcorn

INGREDIENTS: Popcorn, corn oil, Cheddar cheese.

NUTRITION PER SERVING: ½ ounce serving; 90 calories; 1 g protein; 7 g carbohydrate; 6 g fat; 140 mg sodium.

OTHER REPLACEMENTS: Borden Wise Choice Premium Lightly Salted Popcorn; Laura Scudder's Popcorn; Laura Scudder's Popcorn with White Cheddar Cheese.

BE ON THE LOOKOUT FOR: Maizie's Gourmet Popcorn.

MICROWAVE POPCORN

PRODUCT: Betty Crocker Pop Secret Microwave Popcorn

INGREDIENTS: Popcorn, partially hydrogenated soybean oil, salt, TBHQ, citric acid.

NUTRITION PER SERVING: 3 cups popped serving; 120 calories; 2 g protein; 13 g carbohydrate; 8 g* fat; 250 mg sodium.

PRODUCTS TO REPLACE: Most major brands, including: Jolly Time Microwave Popcorn; Planters Premium Select Microwave Popcorn.

REPLACEMENT: Orville Redenbacher's Gourmet Natural Flavor Microwave Popping Corn

INGREDIENTS: Popcorn, partially hydrogenated soybean oil, salt, natural flavors.

NUTRITION PER SERVING: 3 cups popped serving; 100 calories; 2 g protein; 13 g carbohydrate; 6 g fat; 350 mg sodium.

OTHER REPLACEMENTS: Newman's Own Lightly Salted Old Style Picture Show Microwave Popcorn.

RAISINS

PRODUCT: Sun-Maid Golden Raisins

INGREDIENTS: Raisins, sulfur dioxide.

NUTRITION PER SERVING: ½ cup serving; 260 calories; 3 g protein; 68 g carbohydrate; 0 g fat; less than 10 mg sodium.

REPLACEMENT: Dole Raisins, California Seedless

INGREDIENTS: Raisins

NUTRITION PER SERVING: ½ ounce serving; 42 calories; 0 g protein; 11 g carbohydrate; 4 mg sodium.

OTHER REPLACEMENTS: Del Monte Raisins; Sun-Maid Sun-Dried Raisins.

NUTS: PEANUTS

PRODUCT: Planters Honey Roasted Peanuts

INGREDIENTS: Peanuts, sugar, honey, corn syrup, salt, xanthan gum, peanut and/or cottonseed oil.

NUTRITION PER SERVING: 1 ounce serving; 170 calories; 6 g protein; 8 g carbohydrate; 13 g* fat; 160 mg sodium.

PRODUCTS TO REPLACE: All major honey-roasted brands.

REPLACEMENT: Planters Salted Peanuts

INGREDIENTS: Peanuts, peanut and/or cottonseed oil, salt.

NUTRITION PER SERVING: 1 ounce serving; 170 calories; 7 g protein; 5 g carbohydrate; 14 g* fat; 110 mg sodium.

OTHER REPLACEMENTS: Azar nuts—cashews, chopped peanut topping, peanuts, pecans, walnuts.

NUTS: ALMONDS

PRODUCT: Blue Diamond Smokehouse Almonds

INGREDIENTS: Almonds, almond oil and/or safflower oil, salt, maltodextrin, natural hickory flavor, yeast, hydrolyzed vegetable protein, natural flavorings.

NUTRITION PER SERVING: 1 ounce serving; 150 calories; 7 g protein; 4 g carbohydrate; 14 g* fat, 170 mg sodium.

REPLACEMENT: Blue Diamond Blanched Almonds

INGREDIENTS: Almonds, vegetable oil (almond, safflower), salt.

NUTRITION PER SERVING: 1 ounce serving; 150 calories; 7 g protein; 4 g carbohydrate; 14 g* fat; 80 mg sodium.

OTHER REPLACEMENTS: Azar almonds.

CANDY

All major brands of candy are made with sugar or refined sweeteners. However, there can be a big difference after that. Some brands also use more refined sweeteners than others as well as lots of artificial ingredients and preservatives. The comparisons that follow point out the differences between major brands.

PRODUCT: M & M's Plain Chocolate Candies

INGREDIENTS: Milk chocolate (sugar, milk, chocolate, cocoa butter, lecithin, salt, artificial flavors), sugar, cornstarch, corn syrup, gum acacia, artificial colors (including FD&C Yellow No. 5), dextrin.

NUTRITION PER SERVING: 1.69 ounce serving; 240 calories; 3 g protein; 33 g carbohydrate; 10 g fat; 150 mg sodium.

PRODUCTS TO REPLACE: Other brands with artificial ingredients or preservatives, including: M & M's Peanut Chocolate Candies.

REPLACEMENT: Hershey's Kisses

INGREDIENTS: Milk chocolate (sugar, cocoa butter, milk, chocolate, soy lecithin).

NUTRITION PER SERVING: 6 kiss serving; 150 calories; 2 g protein; 16 g carbohydrate; 9 g fat; 25 mg sodium.

OTHER REPLACEMENTS: If you're looking for a sweet treat without lots of additives, you might want to try a handful of Nestlé Semi-Sweet Morsels. They are comparable in ingredients to Hershey's Kisses. Reese's Peanut Butter Cups also have no artificial ingredients or preservatives.

PRODUCT: Mars Milky Way Bar

INGREDIENTS: Milk chocolate (sugar, milk, cocoa butter, chocolate, lecithin, artificial and natural flavors), corn syrup, sugar, milk, partially hydrogenated vegetable oil, malted milk (malted barley flour, milk, baking soda, salt), butter, cocoa, salt, egg whites, soy protein, artificial flavor.

NUTRITION PER SERVING: 1 bar serving; 270 calories; 3 g protein; 41 g carbohydrate; 10 g fat; 80 mg sodium.

PRODUCTS TO REPLACE: All brands with artificial ingredients or preservatives, including: Mars Snickers bar; Mars Three Musketeers bar.

REPLACEMENT: Nestlé Crunch Bar

INGREDIENTS: Milk chocolate (sugar, fresh whole milk, cocoa butter, chocolate, lecithin, vanilla), crisped rice.

NUTRITION PER SERVING: 1 bar serving; 160 calories; 2 g protein; 19 g carbohydrate; 8 g fat; 50 mg sodium.

OTHER REPLACEMENTS: Estee chocolate bars; Hershey's Milk Chocolate with Almonds bar.

PRODUCT: Crunch 'n Munch Buttery Toffee Popcorn with Peanuts

INGREDIENTS: Sugar, corn syrup, peanuts, popcorn, butter, margarine (liquid soybean oil, partially hydrogenated soybean oil, water, salt, sweet dairy whey, lecithin, mono- and diglycerides), sodium benzoate, artificial butter flavor, carotene, vitamin A palmitate, salt, lecithin, baking soda.

NUTRITION PER SERVING: 1 ounce serving; 190 calories; 2 g protein; 24 g carbohydrate; 5 g fat; 120 mg sodium.

PRODUCTS TO REPLACE: Screaming Yellow Zonkers Crispy Light Glazed Popcorn and Nuts.

REPLACEMENT: Cracker Jack

INGREDIENTS: Sugar, corn syrup, popcorn, molasses, corn oil, salt, soy lecithin.

NUTRITION PER SERVING: 1 ounce serving; 120 calories; 2 g protein; 22 g carbohydrate; 3 g fat; 85 mg sodium.

BE ON THE LOOKOUT FOR: Kashi Brittles—Sesame Maple.

DESSERTS: ICE CREAM-FROZEN YOGURT/FROZEN DESSERT BARS/GELATIN/ PACKAGED CAKES AND DESSERTS/BAKING MIXES

ICE CREAM-FROZEN YOGURT

All major brands of ice cream and frozen yogurt—regular or "light"—contain refined sweeteners or artificial sweeteners. However, many brands also add lots of fat, artificial ingredients, and preservatives. In the first comparison, see how a simple, natural, and delicious change can tremendously cut calories and fat. The second comparison shows how to leave lots of artificial ingredients and chemicals behind.

PRODUCT: Häagen-Dazs Vanilla Swiss Almond Ice Cream

INGREDIENTS: Cream, skim milk, sugar, chocolate-coated almonds (roasted almonds, sugar, chocolate liqueur, cocoa butter), egg yolks, vanilla.

NUTRITION PER SERVING: 4 fluid ounce serving; 290 calories; 5 g protein; 24 g carbohydrate; 19 g* fat; 55 mg sodium.

PRODUCTS TO REPLACE: All other high-fat ice creams.

REPLACEMENT: Häagen-Dazs Vanilla Almond Crunch Frozen Yogurt

INGREDIENTS: Skim milk, sugar, corn syrup, almond crunch (almonds, sugar, butter, corn syrup, salt), cream, egg yolk, vanilla, yogurt cultures.

NUTRITION PER SERVING: 3 fluid ounce serving; 150 calories; 5 g protein; 22 g carbohydrate; 5 g fat; 65 mg sodium.

OTHER REPLACEMENTS: All other frozen yogurts that contain no artificial ingredients or preservatives, including all flavors of Häagen-Dazs frozen yogurt.

PRODUCT: Weight Watchers Grand Collection Vanilla Premium Ice Milk

INGREDIENTS: Milk, sugar, nonfat dry milk, corn syrup, cream, microcrystalline cellulose, mono- and diglycerides, natural and artificial flavor, sodium carboxymethylcellulose, guar gum, locust bean gum, polysorbate 80, artificial color, including FD&C Yellow No. 5 and No. 6, carageenan, salt.

NUTRITION PER SERVING: 3 fluid ounce serving; 100 calories; 3 g protein; 16 g carbohydrate; 3 g fat; 75 mg sodium.

PRODUCTS TO REPLACE: All ice milks or frozen yogurts that contain artificial ingredients and preservatives.

REPLACEMENT: Häagen-Dazs Vanilla Frozen Yogurt

INGREDIENTS: Skim milk, sugar, corn syrup, cream, egg yolk, vanilla, yogurt cultures.

NUTRITION PER SERVING: 3 fluid ounce serving; 130 calories; 5 g protein; 20 g carbohydrate; 3 g fat; 40 mg sodium.

OTHER REPLACEMENTS: Any frozen yogurt or ice milk with no artificial ingredients or preservatives.

FROZEN DESSERT BARS

PRODUCT: Welch's Fruit Juice Bars, Assorted Flavors

INGREDIENTS: Grape bar: Water, grape juice from concentrate, sugar, natural flavor, citric acid, guar gum, ascorbic acid. Strawberry bar: Water, white grape juice from concentrate, sugar, strawberry puree from concentrate, guar gum, citric acid, natural and artificial strawberry flavors, ascorbic acid, artificial color. Raspberry bar: Water, white grape juice from concentrate, sugar, raspberry juice from concentrate, guar gum, citric acid, grape color extract, natural and artificial flavors, ascorbic acid, artificial color.

NUTRITION PER SERVING: 1 bar serving; 45 calories; 0 g protein; 11 g carbohydrate; 0 g fat; 0 g sodium.

PRODUCTS TO REPLACE: All major brands containing refined or artificial sweeteners, including: Crystal Light Bars; Disney Pops; Flinstones Push-Up Sherbet Treats; Frozfruit varieties; Knudsen PushUps; Popsicle All Natural Ice Pops; Weight Watchers Sugar Free Orange Vanilla Treat; Welch's No Sugar Added Fruit Juice Bars.

REPLACEMENT: Dole Sun Tops Real Fruit Juice Bars

> INGREDIENTS: Fruit punch bars: white grape, pineapple, orange and cherry juices from concentrates, natural flavors, locust bean and guar gums, turmeric extract.

> NUTRITION PER SERVING: 1 bar serving; 40 calories; less than 1 g protein; 9 g carbohydrate; less than 1 g fat; 5 mg sodium.

> *BE ON THE LOOKOUT FOR:* Ferraro's Natural Juice Sticks—Apple, Boysenberry, Peach.

GELATIN

All major brands of flavored gelatin contain sugar or artificial sweeteners, preservatives, and artificial ingredients. Recommendation: Use sparingly or, as in the comparison below, buy a natural plain gelatin and add your own fruit or juice according to package directions.

PRODUCT: Orange Jell-O Gelatin Dessert

> INGREDIENTS: Sugar, gelatin, adipic acid, disodium phosphate, fumaric acid, artificial color, natural flavor, BHA, artificial flavor.

> NUTRITION PER SERVING: ½ cup serving; 80 calories; 2 g protein; 19 g carbohydrate; 0 g fat, 50 mg sodium.

> PRODUCTS TO REPLACE: All major brands, including: Jell-O—all varieties; Royal Gelatin—all varieties.

REPLACEMENT: Knox Natural Gelatine

> INGREDIENTS: Gelatin. (For fruit gelatin, add 2 cups fruit juice.)

> NUTRITION PER SERVING: 1 envelope serving; 25 calories; 6 g protein; 0 g carbohydrate; 0 g fat; 10 mg sodium.

PACKAGED CAKES AND DESSERTS: APPLE CRISP

All major brands of packaged cakes and desserts—regular, light, or low-fat—contain refined sweeteners or artificial sweeteners. But the difference from there can be startling. Most brands contain many artificial ingredients, chemicals, and preservatives. But, as the comparisons that follow show, a few brands use many fewer such additives.

PRODUCT: Sarah Lee Lights Apple Crisp Cake (in freezer section; sold as single serving or larger)

INGREDIENTS: Apples, sugar, water, corn syrup, enriched bleached flour (malted barley flour, niacin, iron, thiamine mononitrate, riboflavin), skim milk, egg whites, partially hydrogenated vegetable oil (soybean and cottonseed oils), modified food starch, pea fiber, polydextrose, lemon juice, propylene glycol alginate, xanthan gum, propylene glycol monoester, cinnamon, salt, citric acid, mono- and digylcerides, polyglycerol esters of fatty acids, potassium bicarbonate, glucono delta lactone, vanilla, cellulose gum, whole eggs, annatto and turmeric extracts, carob bean gum, honey, flavors, calcium carageenan, ferric phosphate, lemon oil, vitamin A palmitate, thiamine mononitrate, riboflavin.

NUTRITION PER SERVING: 3 ounce serving; 150 calories; 1 g protein; 31 g carbohydrate; 2 g fat; 130 mg sodium.

PRODUCTS TO REPLACE: All major brands containing artificial ingredients or preservatives, including: Dolly Madison; Drake; Hostess; Hostess Light; Pillsbury's Best Danishes; Sarah Lee.

REPLACEMENT: Pepperidge Farm Apple Crisp (in freezer section; sold as single serving or larger)

INGREDIENTS: Apples, milk, corn syrup, sugar, water, unbleached wheat flour, egg yolks, modified food starch, partially hydrogenated vegetable shortening, nonfat milk, invert syrup, butter, spices, cornstarch, salt, vanilla extract, egg whites, baking soda.

NUTRITION PER SERVING: 4.75 ounce serving; 250 calories; 2 g protein; 43 g carbohydrate; 8 g fat; 130 mg sodium.

OTHER REPLACEMENTS: Other brands containing few additives and no artificial ingredients, including: Pepperidge Farm Frozen Blueberry Turnovers.

PACKAGED CAKES AND DESSERTS: BROWNIES

PRODUCT: Weight Watchers Chocolate Brownie (in freezer section)

INGREDIENTS: Apple juice concentrate, eggs, egg whites, fructose, polydextrose, chocolate chips (sugar, chocolate liqueur, cocoa butter, lecithin, salt, artificial flavor), enriched flour (niacin, iron, thiamine mononitrate, riboflavin), powdered cellulose, cocoa powder, alkali, sugar, calcium sodium casseinate, mono- and diglycerides, walnuts, natural and artificial flavor, sodium bicarbonate, potassium bicarbonate, sodium saccharin, cellulose gum.

NUTRITION PER SERVING: 1.25 ounce serving; 100 calories; 3 g protein; 16 g carbohydrate; 3 g fat; 150 mg sodium.

REPLACEMENT: Pepperidge Farm Hot Fudge Brownie (in freezer section)

INGREDIENTS: Sugar, unbleached wheat flour, butter, whole eggs, light cream, chocolate liqueur, walnuts, cocoa, alkali, dextrose, water, corn syrup, invert syrup, partially hydrogenated vegetable shortening, vanilla extract, natural flavoring, gelatin.

NUTRITION PER SERVING: 1 ounce serving; 133 calories; 1 g protein; 17 g carbohydrate; 6 g fat; 80 mg sodium.

BAKING MIXES

All major brands of cake and other baking mixes contain refined or artificial sweeteners and lots of artificial ingredients, chemicals, and preservatives. Recommendation: Use sparingly. However, we found a muffin mix that does compare favorably to another brand.

PRODUCT: Betty Crocker Corn Muffin Mix

INGREDIENTS: Enriched bleached flour, enriched degermed yellow cornmeal, vegetable shortening, BHA, BHT, dextrose (corn syrup), sugar, baking soda, sodium aluminum phosphate, monocalcium phosphate, salt, wheat starch.

NUTRITION PER SERVING: 1 muffin serving; 160 calories; 3 g protein; 25 g carbohydrate; 5 g fat; 315 mg sodium.

PRODUCTS TO REPLACE: All major brands, including Duncan Hines, Jiffy Corn Muffin Mix.

REPLACEMENT: Pepperidge Farm Old Fashioned Corn Muffin Mix

INGREDIENTS: Unbleached enriched flour, nonfat milk, yellow cornmeal, sugar, eggs, partially hydrogenated soybean oil, baking soda, modified food starch, salt.

NUTRITION PER SERVING: 1 muffin serving; 180 calories; 3 g protein; 27 g carbohydrate; 7 g fat; 259 mg sodium.

BE ON THE LOOKOUT FOR: Fearn cake and muffin mixes.

BABY FOOD: CEREAL/ JUICE/MAIN DISH

BABY FOOD: CEREAL

All major brands of baby cereal are enriched, but they have no added sugar. Any choice in this category would be a good one.

BE ON THE LOOKOUT FOR: Familia Swiss Baby Cereal. This brand is being introduced in supermarkets nationally. It is not enriched. Instead it uses four types of whole grains.

BABY FOOD: JUICE

Most baby juices are pure juice, but some products have added sugar and additives.

PRODUCT: Gerber Apple Juice with Lowfat Yogurt

INGREDIENTS: Apple juice from concentrate, lowfat yogurt (cultured lowfat milk, nonfat dry milk, gelatin, citrus pectin), sugar, citrus pectin, vitamin C, citric acid.

NUTRITION PER SERVING: 4 ounce serving; 100 calories; 3 g protein; 19 g carbohydrate; 1 g fat; 45 mg sodium.

PRODUCTS TO REPLACE: Any other brands containing refined or artificial sweeteners or preservatives, including: Gerber Baby Juices—Banana Juice Medley with Lowfat Yogurt, Mixed Fruit Juice with Lowfat Yogurt, Pear-Peach Juice with Lowfat Yogurt.

REPLACEMENT: Gerber Apple Juice

INGREDIENTS: Apple juice, vitamin C.

NUTRITION PER SERVING: 4.2 ounce serving; 60 calories; 0 g protein; 15 g carbohydrate; 0 g fat; 0 mg sodium.

OTHER REPLACEMENTS: Beech-Nut Stages Real Juice—Apple Cranberry, Mixed Fruit; Gerber juices—Apple-Banana, Apple-Cherry, Mixed Fruit, Pear; Heinz baby juices—Apple, Apple-Cherry.

BABY FOOD: MAIN DISH

Most baby/toddler main dishes are just strained versions of pure foods. However, some on the market add sugar or other additives.

PRODUCT: Gerber Macaroni Alphabets with Beef and Tomato Sauce

INGREDIENTS: Water, tomato puree, beef (beef, chopped and formed, salt, onion powder), enriched macaroni, rice flour, peas, corn, wheat flour, potato starch, sugar, salt, onion powder, soybean oil, extract of celery, pepper.

NUTRITION PER SERVING: 6.25 ounce serving; 140 calories; 7 g protein; 20 g carbohydrate; 4 g fat; 370 mg sodium.

PRODUCTS TO REPLACE: Any other brands containing sugar or additives, including: Gerber Chicken Stick finger food for toddlers.

REPLACEMENT: Beech-Nut Stages Turkey Rice Dinner

INGREDIENTS: Water, carrots, turkey, peas, rice starch, rice flour, long grain rice, onion powder, celery seed.

NUTRITION PER SERVING: 6 ounce serving; 90 calories; 3 g protein; 14 g carbohydrate; 3 g fat; 65 mg sodium.

OTHER REPLACEMENTS: All entrées containing no sugar or additives, including: Beech-Nut Stages—Vegetable Chicken Dinner; Gerber Chunky Vegetables and Chicken for Toddlers; Gerber Junior—Beef, Ham, Strained Chicken, Strained Lamb; Gerber Second Foods—Beef, Turkey, Veal.

GLOSSARY

Assume that additives mentioned have been classified by the FDA as GRAS (Generally Recognized as Safe)—but remember, as noted in Chapter 3, that the government never gives additives permanent approval. Approved additives are continually reviewed by the FDA and FSIS to assess whether approvals should be modified or withdrawn, but additives remain in the food supply while testing is conducted. For further information on the three thousand additives in our foods, consult an additive dictionary, (some of which are mentioned in the bibliography).

Acetic acid (also referred to on some food labels as sodium diacetyl) The substance in vinegar that supplies its taste and odor. Manufacturers, who mainly produce the substance chemically from alcohol and acetaldehyde, use it as a flavoring, preservative, or a way to give acidity to many foods. Much of the acetic acid made in the United States is used in the manufacture of plastic. Much higher concentrations of acetic acid than is used in foods can corrode the digestive tract.

Adipic acid Occurs naturally in small amounts in beet juice and butter. Adipic acid used commercially is produced synthetically. It is used in beverages and candies to enhance flavor, control acidity, lighten texture of baked goods, and as a preservative. Also used in the manufacture of plastics and nylons.

Alkali A substance that neutralizes acids.

Aluminum sulfate (and other aluminum compounds) The most abundant metallic element in the earth's crust. Small amounts appear in many foods. Aluminum sulfate is a firming agent that is a white powder used in producing pickles and as a modifier in food starch used in many food products. Other aluminum compounds are used as leavening agents in bread products. Kidney patients may suffer adverse effects from aluminum and should consult physicians regarding avoiding such additives. Because of a body of studies, and the recent possible links of aluminum compounds to diseases like Alzheimer's, many organizations raise questions about the use of aluminum compounds. Aluminum sulfate is also used in tanning leather, sizing paper, waterproofing for antiperspirants, agricultural pesticides and detergents.

Ammonium sulfate (and other ammonium compounds) Used as a yeast-food dough conditioner as well as in bakery products. Those with kidney or liver problems may be affected. Industrially used in fireproofing fabrics, tanning and fertilizers.

Annatto (extract and seed) From a tropical tree, annatto is used as a vegetable dye and spice flavoring in many products.

Artificial colors Originally, artificial colors were produced by heating coal and converting it to impure forms. Thus they are also known as coal tar dyes. Currently produced from chemicals purer than those originating from coal, they are used often in foods, cosmetics, and fabrics. Artificial colors are controversial. They are constantly being scrutinized by the FDA. Over the years, certain strains of colors have been withdrawn because of possible links to cancer.

Artificial flavors When artificial is used to describe any additive, it means that the additive has no counterpart and is not duplicated in nature.

Ascorbic acid Vitamin C manufactured as a preservative.

Aspartame Called NutraSweet under a patent arrangement in the United States. (See Chapter 3.)

Autolyzed yeast or yeast autolyzates A by-product of brewing yeast; approved as GRAS based on current information, but the FDA has stated that not enough information was available so tests are still being conducted.

Beet powder Vegetable dye used as food coloring.

Benzoate of soda (sodium benzoate) A preservative, it is a white odorless powder used in soft drinks, margarine, jams, and jellies. Also used in ice to cool fish, and in human liver tests. Studies have shown that it can cause intestinal upset and allergic reaction. Food may only contain .1 percent of this additive.

Beta carotene From the vitamin A family, a nontoxic substance used to color foods.

BHA (Butylated hydroxyanisole) A controversial preservative used in many products; a white, waxy solid. The liver detoxifies BHA, and it has been shown to affect the liver and kidney. Since uncertainties exist, tests are still being conducted.

BHT (Butylated hydroxytoluene) Used in many foods to retard rancidity and, like BHA, is controversial. It has caused allergic reactions. Mice fed large amounts of this substance gave birth to offspring with chemical changes in their brains. There are still questions regarding the effect of BHT on women taking oral contraceptives. Tests continue.

Bleaching A chemical process often used to age and mature dough.

Bromate Used to mature dough. High doses have caused poisoning of children and a food poisoning outbreak in New Zealand.

Caffeine (Guaranine; Methyltheobromine; Theine; Trimethylxanthine) An odorless white powder that has a bitter taste. Caffeine is a drug that is classified medically as a poison. Morphine and strychnine are in the same family. (See also Chapter 3.)

Calcium carbonate A white food dye that occurs naturally in rocks and is used in wine and ice cream. All litters of rodents fed varying amounts of calcium carbonate were lower in number and weight. Mortality also increased and some mice were born with enlarged hearts. Human ulcer patients were tested with it at 150 times the amount used in foods. Many patients experienced nausea and dizziness.

Calcium casseinate A protein from cow's milk used in dairy products and some diet foods. Industrially, also used in the manufacture of paint and plastic.

Calcium chloride A firming agent used in pie mixes, jellies and as an additive in some cheeses. Industrially, used in automobile antifreeze, for dust control on unpaved roads, and to preserve wood. As a food additive, has been shown to cause stomach upset and heart irregularities.

Calcium disodium EDTA A preservative used for flavor retention in many foods. Has been shown to cause kidney problems, cramps, and blood in the urine. It is currently under priority for FDA testing.

Caramel coloring A chemical group produced by heating carbohydrates; burnt sugar. The process of making caramel coloring has been linked to blood toxicity in rats.

Carob bean gum A food thickener and stabilizer from the carob plant used in ice cream, candy, dressings, jellies and other foods. Testing of this additive continues.

Carageenan A glue-like substance used as a food emulsifer. High dosages have been shown to cause cancer to develop after two years in rats. Tests continue.

Citric acid Used in many foods, a by-product of fermentation of crude sugars. A varied additive with many uses.

Corn syrup (dextrose) Used in flavorings for beverages and baked goods, cereals, cheeses, and many other foods. Also used for envelopes, tapes, and stamps. Has been shown to cause allergies in some people.

Dipotassium phosphate A buffering agent used in cheese and nondairy coffee creamers. Also used in automobile antifreeze.

Disodium guanylate The salt of guanylic acid that is used as a flavor enhancer, like monosodium glutamate.

Disodium inosinate A flavor enhancer.

Ferrous sulfate An iron source added to foods as well as being used as a wood preserver and weed killer.

Fumaric acid White and odorless, it is prepared industrially from many plants and used as a leavening agent or a dry acid in food products.

Glycerin (Glycerol) A by-product when soaps and fatty acids are manufactured, it's a sweet-tasting substance that's used as a body-giving agent and plasticizer in foods. Also used in perfume and in suppositories for constipation.

Glycerol ester of wood rosin Used in chewing gum and as a beverage stabilizer; made from wood rosin and glycerin.

Guar gum A powder derived from Indian plants that is used in many food products. It is also used as a bulk laxative and to treat ulcers.

High fructose corn syrup Corn syrup that is chemically altered to change its glucose to fructose. Used in soft drinks and many other products. (See also Chapter 4.)

Hydrogenation The adding of hydrogen gas under high pressure to liquid oils. Process used in manufacture of margarine and other products. Tests have recently shown that hydrogenated foods may cause the body to manufacture cholesterol.

Hydrolyzed vegetable protein A flavor enhancer that contains monosodium glutamate. Some of its components have been shown to affect growth, yet it is used in some baby foods. The FDA advisory boards have asked that testing in relation to its effect on children continue.

Invert sugar An equal mixture of glucose and fructose.

Lactic acid A bacterial acid that occurs in sour milk and is used in many foods.

Lecithin Isolated from eggs, corn and egg yolks and used as a preservative in cereals, bread, candy, and many other foods.

Malt extract Taken from germinated, heated and then dried barley.

Methionine An essential amino acid used in cooking oil to make chips, soups, and other foods taste fresher. Considered GRAS, but the FDA has requested further study.

Modified food starch Starch that has been changed chemically and added to foods; used in some baby foods because it is easy to digest. Effect on children and their ability to handle the chemicals are unknown. Tests continue.

Monosodium glutamate (MSG) A natural flavor enhancer, to which some people have an allergic reaction. MSG has been shown to cause brain damage in young rodents and other animals. Female animals treated with it had fewer and smaller litters, and male fertility was affected. It has been removed from baby products. Tests continue.

Natural flavors Flavors derived from a natural, rather than an artificial, source. (See also Chapter 4.)

Oleoresin Oil and resin extracted from a plant substance through use of alcohol or ether. Used in foods for color or flavor.

Olestra A fake fat developed by Procter and Gamble that is under review by the FDA.

Petrolatum (petroleum jelly) Sealant and coating for some foods. It is thought that it is not digested, but it may cause a slight laxative effect.

Phosphoric acid Obtained from phosphate rock, it is used in many products, including soft drinks.

Polysorbate 60 An emulsifier and disperser of flavor. Testing continues.

Potassium bromate Adds sponge-like qualities to breads. Tests have shown it to be a possible carcinogen.

Propylene glycol monostearate A wax that is used in foods as a dough conditioner and a lubricating agent. In large doses, has been shown to cause kidney and nervous system problems.

Pyridoxine hydrochloride Vitamin B_6.

Riboflavin A factor in vitamin B-complex; added to many enriched foods.

Saccharin An artificial sweetener that is 300 times sweeter than sugar. Products using it must carry a warning that it has possibly caused cancer in laboratory animals.

Sodium citrate An emulsifier used in ice cream, processed cheese and many other products. Also used to control acidity in food products. Can affect the effectiveness of drugs in the body.

Sodium compounds Perform many different functions in foods, from preservatives, to bleaching agents, to flavor enhancers. However, all add sodium to the diet. Examples: Sodium acid pyrophophate, sodium alginate, sodium aluminum diglycerides, sodium aluminum phosphate, sodium aluminum sulfate, sodium ascorbate, sodium benzoate, sodium bicarbonate, sodium bisulfite, sodium carbonate, sodium casseinate, sodium diacetyl, sodium erthorbate, sodium metabisulfite, sodium nitrate, sodium phosphate.

Sodium sulfite Because it has caused dangerous allergic reactions in some people, use has been halted in most products, but it is still used in wines and a few other products.

Sorbic acid Originally from plants but also created chemically by food manufacturers. Used as a preservative in foods as well as cosmetics. When large doses were injected into animals, cancer was caused.

Sorbitol A sweet powder used as a sugar substitute for diabetics and as a food stabilizer. Also used in tobacco, leather, antifreeze, and writing inks. Can cause diarrhea, and may alter the absorption of drugs in the body.

Sucrose The same as sugar, cane sugar, and beet sugar. (See also Chapter 4.)

Sulfur dioxide The gas formed when sulfur burns; used to preserve dried fruits and in many other foods. The gas itself is poisonous and irritating. When concentrated and inhaled, it has caused death.

TBHQ (Tertiary Butylhydroquinone) A controversial preservative that was put on the market after much pushing by food manufacturers. Larger doses than those currently used in foods have caused problems ranging from nausea to death.

TATCA (Trialkoxytricarballylate) An oil-like fake fat with no calories developed by CPC International.

Titanium dioxide A pigment that occurs in minerals and is used for food coloring.

Whey The watery part of milk that is left after separation when cheese is made.

Xanthan gum A gum produced by the bacteria present in the fermenting of corn sugar; products may pour more easily when it is used.

Zinc oxide Zinc metal produces zinc oxide, which is added to food as a nutrient. When ingested on its own, it has caused nausea and vomiting.

BIBLIOGRAPHY

*Freydberg, Nicholas and Willis Gortner. *The Food Additives Book*. New York: Bantam, 1982.

*Jacobson, Michael. *The Complete Eater's Digest and Nutrition Scoreboard: The Consumer's Factbook of Food Additives and Healthful Eating*. New York: Doubleday, 1985.

Stern, Bert, Lawrence Chilnick, and Lynn Sonberg. *The Food Book: The Complete Guide to the Most Popular Brand Name Foods in the United States*. New York: Dell, 1989.

*Winter, Ruth. *A Consumer's Dictionary of Food Additives*. New York: Crown, 1984.

*Recommended further reading for those interested in dictionaries of food additives.

INDEX